Live Di...
Ps 116:8
Dianne

Please!

23 118-8-9

Live Delivered!

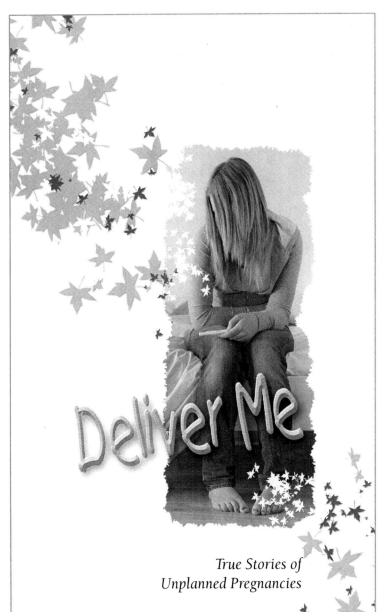

Deliver Me

*True Stories of
Unplanned Pregnancies*

*Compiled and Edited
by Dianne E. Butts*

ISBN 978-0-9831649-0-6

Published by
Connections Press
Pueblo, Colorado

Stories Compiled & Edited By
Dianne E. Butts

Book Edited By
Marjorie Vawter

*Asterisks beside a person's name throughout this book indicate the
name has been changed to protect the privacy of the individual.*

Cover and Interior Design
J. L. Hardesty

Printed in the USA

For all the unnamed people who give so generously
of their hearts, time, and resources
to help those who have experienced
an unplanned or unwanted pregnancy.
May God bless you abundantly.

Table of Contents

Table of Contents

Table of Contents

Table of Contents

Acknowledgements

It is amazing to sit down to write these acknowledgements and realize how many people were involved in the making of this book and how many people there are who, if it weren't for them, this book would not exist.

I would like to thank all those who contributed their stories. Many are named in these pages. Others asked not to be named for confidentiality, but the Lord knows who you are. May He bless all of you for sharing your stories. It was my deep desire to help you write your stories in order to share their power with anyone and everyone who would grace us with their time and read these pages. You've made my dream come true. It has been my honor and privilege to work with each of you, and to give you an opportunity to share the power in your stories through writing and producing this book. But I'm only the writer. You lived it. Obviously without your willingness to share your story, this book would not exist.

I also wish to acknowledge and thank everyone—and there were many of you, too many to remember let alone name—who talked with me and encouraged me over the years I put this book together. You have helped me in ways beyond what I can put into words. Special thanks to my writing "Barnabas" group—Gayle Gresham, LaRose Karr, Tanya Warrington, and Marlene Depler—for your help, expertise, prayers, support, and encouragement.

I thank all of those who have supported this project with your prayers. If I tried to name all those who have prayed for this book, I would certainly make a miserable mess of that. There are too many of you! But as I neared completion of the book, the special prayer team became Bonnie Castillo, Margi Wilson, and the wonderful intercessory prayer group at the First Presbyterian Church in Lamar, Colorado: Nadine McClung, Caryol Heckman, Theresa Eisenhouer, Marjorie Wyatt, and Pat Gillespie. Without your prayers, I don't believe this book would exist.

I thank Marlene Bagnull for all the training I've received at her Colorado Christian Writers Conferences, for teaching me so much about publishing, as well as for her encouragement over the many years I've known her.

Special thanks to my attorney, Linda McMillan, who does her best to keep me out of trouble . . . and then helps me when I get into trouble anyway. Your generous help has blessed me beyond what I can express and I'm very, very grateful to you. Without your help in many ways, I would not have been able to bring this book into existence.

Thanks to Margie Vawter, my wonderful editor (and friend) who helped me polish the manuscript to the best we could make it. And to Shelley Ring whose marketing expertise has been extremely helpful.

I would especially like to thank and acknowledge Jo Hardesty Lauter, whose incredibly generous offer to help me with the book's cover and interior design suddenly made this whole project possible. Without you, Jo, this book would not exist.

Thanks to my wonderful, supportive husband, Hal. Without your constant support and encouragement this book wouldn't exist.

I also thank my Lord Jesus Christ who ultimately brought me each of the stories in this book as well as the means to produce the book. Without Your love, mercy, atoning sacrifice, and forgiveness none of these stories or this book would exist. May it bring people to know You as You truly are and bring You glory.

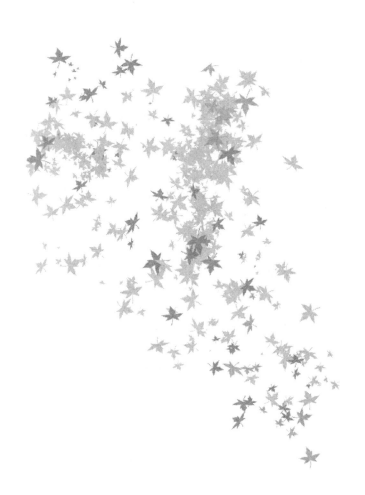

I love the LORD,
for he heard my voice; he heard my cry for mercy.
Because he turned his ear to me,
I will call on him as long as I live.
The cords of death entangled me,
the anguish of the grave came upon me;
I was overcome by trouble and sorrow.
Then I called on the name of the LORD:
"O LORD, save me!"
The LORD is gracious and righteous;
our God is full of compassion.
The LORD protects the simplehearted;
when I was in great need, he saved me.
Be at rest once more, O my soul,
for the LORD has been good to you.
For you, O LORD, have delivered my
soul from death, my eyes from tears,
my feet from stumbling, that I may
walk before the LORD in the land of the living. . . .
How can I repay the LORD for all his goodness to me?
I will lift up the cup of salvation
and call on the name of the LORD. . . .
You have freed me from my chains.

PSALM 116:1–9, 12–13, 16 NIV

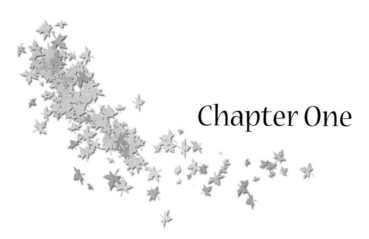

Chapter One

Who Faces Unplanned Pregnancy?

I was overcome by trouble. Psalm 116:3

We may think those facing unplanned pregnancies are usually unwed teenage girls. But if abortion statistics can give us a glimpse of who faces unplanned pregnancy, fewer than one-fifth (18%) of abortions in the United States are obtained by teenagers.[1]

The fact is, women of all childbearing ages—including teenagers, even preteens, as well as women in their thirties and forties—both single and married, face unplanned pregnancy. For every pregnancy, often overlooked is the man involved. And many times the pregnancy affects the entire family of the mother- and father-to-be.

When that pregnancy test shows positive, she must face the many fears and dilemmas that go with an unplanned pregnancy. In the middle of her shock and panic, where can she go for help? Who can she turn to? Women facing an unplanned pregnancy, the man in her life, her parents and siblings, and others touched by her pregnancy can find hope, help, and healing in the stories of those who have gone before, those who have faced an unplanned pregnancy themselves.

How did they handle it? What did they do? Do they have any regrets? Are they pleased with their choices?

About 14% of recent births to women 15 to 44 years of age in 2002 were unwanted at the time of conception.²

*Asterisks next to a person's name throughout this book indicate the name has been changed to protect the privacy of the individual.

For others, there is an unplanned pregnancy in your past. Whether recent or distant in years, you may still feel the many decisions you made and the heartaches you faced at that time in your life. How and where can you find healing? In the stories of those who have gone before.

You may not be the one who experienced the unplanned pregnancy directly. You may be the father of the child, or the parent, sibling, or friend of the woman who faced the unplanned pregnancy. You, also, will find stories in this book that speak to you.

The true stories of those who have been there—like Sandi*² and Vera Cole,* whose stories you'll read in this first chapter—can teach us and help others now facing the same dilemmas. Whether in hindsight these women are pleased with the choices they made, regret them, or fall somewhere in between, we can learn how the choices these women made affected their lives, where they found help, what options and resources they discovered along the way, and how they have recovered from their unplanned pregnancy. Knowing we are not alone and seeing how others have handled the situation, not only helps us, it gives us hope. When we find ourselves in desperate and devastating circumstances, that's what we need: hope and help.

And when we've been through something—however long ago—that remains unhealed, we can also find healing for ourselves in discovering where others found healing.

Below you will meet two women: one young, the other reaching the older end of childbearing age. Each had diverse *circumstances. Each with a story as unique as she is.*

Sandi* was one young woman who needed help. So utterly alone, she had no idea who to turn to for help. But Sandi found the help she needed when she met Phyllis Allen, and her story can help others find the help they need.

When I first saw the young woman standing outside the office window, I tried to ignore her. *She's probably just passing*

"I'm Not Pregnant, But..."

by Phyllis Allen

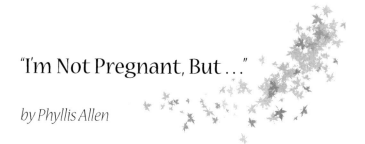

by, I thought. On that rainy Saturday afternoon, PAL—the Pregnancy Assistance League—wasn't open for clients. But I was in the office anyway. As executive director of PAL, I often stayed late or worked weekends to train volunteers or to catch up on the never-ending duties of keeping a pregnancy center running.

But when I glanced up again, she was still standing there, the rain running down her hair and soaking through her baggy navy sweats. I knew something was terribly wrong. She turned and paced back and forth, then returned to stare at the sign on the door again. She never did try the door or even knock, but the look of hopelessness on her face told me this was where she needed to be.

As she started to turn away again, I rushed to the door and jerked it open. "Hi!" I said. "Welcome to PAL! Would you like to come in?"

The young woman stepped past me and stood just inside the door, contemplating the toes of her worn tennis shoes. The twin sisters Dread and Despair accompany many clients to our door, but this one seemed unusually fearful. I closed the door against the cold and offered her some hot chocolate. She nodded gratefully but still didn't speak. *Lord, help me put her fears at ease and find out why You brought her here today,* I prayed silently.

I chatted on about the gray, drizzly day outside, and the girl gradually warmed to the homelike atmosphere of the office. She responded to my questions but wouldn't meet my eyes. Her name was Sandi* and she worked as a horse trainer in a nearby town. She was twenty-two.

I showed her to the counseling room. She slipped into a wooden rocker. She looked completely exhausted. Handing her a clipboard with an intake form, I left her to scour the storage room for towels and blankets. I prayed. I still didn't know why she was here, but I knew God had brought her to this place on this day and I trusted He would accomplish His plan for her.

Returning to the counseling room, I found Sandi doubled up in the rocker—her face pale and her eyes wide with fear. *"Sandi!"* I hurried to her side.

When she'd caught her breath, she confided, "I haven't felt well the last couple weeks. It just keeps getting worse, but I don't have any money to go to a doctor. I feel ten times worse today—and then I heard your radio ad. So I came here. I don't know if you can me help or not."

"So you came for a pregnancy test, then?" I asked.

"No!" she exclaimed. "I'm sure I'm not pregnant! I just thought maybe you could help me. I don't know *what* I was thinking!"

"It's okay." I patted her arm. Her baggy sweats were soaked through and clung to her well-rounded form. A certain fear began nagging my mind. "You know, maybe we could start by eliminating possibilities," I suggested. "You're pretty sure you're not pregnant, but let's do the test so we can rule that out

 18

completely and go on to another possible reason for your illness."

Surprisingly, Sandi seemed satisfied with this plan. I helped her perform the test.

While we waited for the timer to ring, I said, "You indicated on your intake form you didn't know when your last period was. Can you give me an estimate?"

"Not really," she replied. "It's been several months, I think. I fell off a horse and I haven't had one since. I felt okay for a long time. It was no big deal."

When the timer rang, Sandi read the results. She slumped back into the rocking chair and tears began rolling down her cheeks. "Are you *s-s-sure*?" She looked incredulous. "I can't believe it! How could I not know? I can't do this! I can't have a baby!"

"Sandi, this may be difficult, but we can help you through it if you'll let us," I assured her. "Would it be all right if I prayed with you and asked God to help us find an answer to your problem?"

Too overwhelmed to speak, Sandi nodded. I grasped her hands and prayed for God's wisdom. When I opened my eyes, Sandi's tears had stopped, but her face had grown pale again and she was breathless.

"Let's try to pinpoint when you became pregnant," I said, growing more concerned. After a considerable amount of thought and figuring, I stared at the possible due date. It verified that nagging fear I had. This girl was not only pregnant, she was having this baby *now*!

My own astonishment was nothing compared to Sandi's shock when I told her.

She lay down on the couch and I timed her contractions—they were already coming ten minutes apart. But Sandi refused to go to the hospital. She had no money and she didn't want to have this baby!

"Is there someone I can call?" I asked urgently. "Your mother? Your boyfriend?"

Angrily, she shook her head. "I told you I have no one! I haven't spoken to my folks in months. And there is no boyfriend.

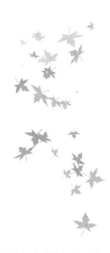

Among recent births:

64% occurred within marriage,

14% occurred within cohabiting unions,

21% to women who were neither married nor cohabiting.[3]

I hardly knew the guy who did this to me!" She sobbed frantically. "No one cares what happens to me—I don't even care anymore!"

"Sandi"—I swallowed back my own fears—"you are not alone. God is with you. He brought you here today because He loves you and He loves your baby. He will help you through this, and I will stay with you. This situation is way beyond your control now . . . but nothing is ever out of God's control. Even if you've never known Him before, you're going to have to trust Him now!"

Biting her lip, Sandi fought back the tears. From that moment on, she accepted responsibility for the baby about to be born.

I started making phone calls. Sandi relaxed between contractions. I knew Medicaid's Baby Care program would cover the hospital expenses, but on Saturday no one was at the local Social Services office. I called the hospital, but they would need a Medicaid number to admit her. Praying, I called a friend who administered the Baby Care program in the county where I lived. Following a hurried explanation, she assured me Sandi and the baby would be eligible, but she would have to be a resident of the county. "When she gets out of the hospital, she's staying with me," I said.

"That works for me," she said. She gave me the Medicaid number and called ahead to the Emergency Room. They'd be expecting us.

The contractions grew stronger, coming every seven minutes. I helped Sandi to my van. "Maybe your family could help you," I suggested as we drove. "New babies have a way of healing old wounds between family members." But Sandi adamantly refused to contact her family.

"What about the baby's father?" I asked. "What do you think his reaction to your pregnancy will be?"

"I have no idea where he even is." She wept. "I know I have no choice about having this baby, but I just can't take care of it! I can't even take care of myself. What kind of mother would I be?"

"Adoption is always a possibility," I suggested. "It's a difficult choice, but it's a loving one." Sandi looked skeptical. "Thousands of couples would give anything to have a baby, but they can't," I reassured her. "You could help choose a family who will love and cherish your baby."

At the ER, medical personnel whisked her off to Maternity. I sat by her bedside. Between paperwork and examinations, we talked. Sandi wanted to place the child for adoption immediately. She didn't want to see the baby, and she would not take it home even temporarily. She also insisted the baby not spend even one day with anyone other than the people who would be the family she could not be.

As an adoptive parent myself, I knew the adoption process could be long and filled with mountains of paperwork. I didn't know if what Sandi asked were even possible. But I admired her determination to do what she thought right for the baby. Holding hands at her bedside, Sandi and I prayed that God would help us find the family that was waiting to make her precious baby their own.

Whenever Sandi could rest, I slipped out into the hall and made frantic phone calls. I called one of PAL's board members for names and numbers of Christian adoption agencies we had worked with. She looked them up with some hesitation. "This isn't following our protocols," she said.

"I know," I said, "but this is the very heart and soul of the ministry we operate." She contacted the other board members to pray for everything going on at the hospital and behind the scenes.

A few calls down the list, I found a live person instead of an answering machine. The adoption counselor listened to my story incredulously. She had adoptive couples standing by on waiting lists. And she agreed to travel the two-hundred miles first thing the next morning to meet with Sandi and commence the process.

I stayed with Sandi throughout her labor and delivery. In the wee hours of the morning, Sandi gave birth to a beautiful, healthy boy. Exhausted but happy, Sandi had transformed at some point during the day from a terrified kid in denial into a mature and responsible young woman seeing to every detail of providing a loving adoptive home for her newborn son.

The adoption counselor arrived and met with Sandi for hours, satisfying any question that Sandi was sure in her decision. Then they began the daunting task of all that paperwork. Later that afternoon, an ecstatic young couple arrived and was introduced to their new son, whom they named Philip.*

Everyone encouraged Sandi to see and hold him, but she would not. "I might change my mind," she confided to me, "and that wouldn't be what is best for Philip."

Sandi stayed with me after leaving the hospital and spent two days recovering physically and emotionally. Then, as suddenly as she'd come into my life, she departed. I've never seen her or heard from her since that day, but many lives were changed forever by her brave and selfless actions. Philip is now nine years old.

The situations of women caught up in unplanned pregnancies are as unique and individual as they are. It's not just young women—

teenagers or preteens—who need help. Older women can also be surprised by an unplanned pregnancy. Here Vera Cole* tells her story of helping a woman in the older childbearing age range.

The first phone call came to my home via the hotline. It was late at night and I was ready to climb into bed after a long day.

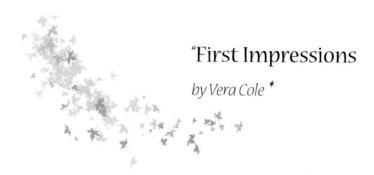

"First Impressions

by Vera Cole *

"Hello. Hotline. May I help you?"

The woman on the other end of the line sounded panicked. "I think I might be pregnant," she said. Her story tumbled out over the phone line, all her fears and doubts thrown at the feet of a complete stranger. We talked until midnight. She called again the next night at the same hour and again the following night. Each time I encouraged her to come into the pregnancy center for an appointment, but she insisted on the anonymity of a phone line.

Casi* was thirty-six years old. Like my younger clients, she was frantic about the possibility of having a baby and taking on all the responsibility it involved. But unlike my teenage clients, this woman had established a lifestyle of sexual activity. She had been sexually intimate with a host of men and had no idea which one might be the father of this child. Some of her partners had been black, others white, still others Hispanic.

She wasn't even sure what color skin this child might have. In addition she faced the mounting pressures of financial debt. She had maxed out all her credit cards. Lawyers had already contacted her about foreclosure on her home.

Night after night she continued to call. I gave her my home phone number so she wouldn't have to talk to a different hotline volunteer each night. I also set boundaries on our relationship . . . no more phone calls after 10:00 p.m.

After weeks of calls, I at last persuaded Casi to make an appointment so that we could meet face-to-face at my office. By

Of all abortions in the United States:

36% occur to non-Hispanic white women

30% occur to non-Hispanic black women,

25% occur to Hispanic women and 9% occur to women of other races. [4]

this time I had created a picture in my mind's eye of this woman. She must be an attractive woman to have so many partners. Her voice projected the image of a strong woman who, though thrown by current circumstances, was by nature confident and in control.

On the day of her appointment, I waited for her to arrive. How could I, a white woman happily married and living in suburbia, relate to a woman from such a vastly different background? Would I be able to establish a connection that would allow me to help her through this crisis?

I peeked into the lobby. There she sat. She was a heavyset woman. Her hair appeared greasy and matted. Streaks of gray had invaded her once-brown locks. Her polyester slacks and tight pink tank top had pulled threads and looked like they had not been washed in weeks. She slumped in the chair. Everything about her screamed vulnerability.

This was the woman who had intimidated me? All my own fears melted as I suddenly focused on her needs instead of my own inadequacies. Here was an injured child who yearned for God's love.

"Casi? I'm Vera. Come on in to my office."

She looked up at me with surprise. "You're Vera? You're nothing like what I pictured."

With an inner smile, I thought, *And you, my dear, are nothing like what I expected!*

Weeks passed and turned into months. Casi decided to carry her child to term. We discussed the pros and cons of adoption. She opted to parent her child because her own father had abandoned her as a child. We put her in touch with legal aid and a solid financial counselor. I shared with her the story of a heavenly Father who would never abandon her.

Almost a year later Casi walked into our center again. She looked down at the infant sleeping in her arms. Brushing a stray hair off the forehead of her child, she said a single word: "Thanks!"

Some women in unplanned pregnancies have families who

support them, others have families who present real challenges. Some clients have no family involved at all. In between the young women like Sandi and the older women like Casi are the vast majority of women who are caught up in a variety of circumstances as unique and individual as they are. But help is available to anyone who wants it. If you are in an unplanned pregnancy, or know someone who is, you can find help and hope. Here are some Resources to help you find the help you need.

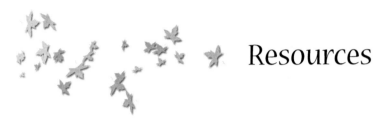 # Resources

Find a caring pregnancy center near you, like Sandi and Casi found. Here are some resources:

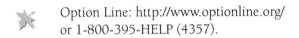 Option Line: http://www.optionline.org/ or 1-800-395-HELP (4357).

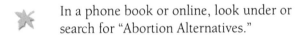 In a phone book or online, look under or search for "Abortion Alternatives."

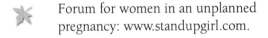 Forum for women in an unplanned pregnancy: www.standupgirl.com.

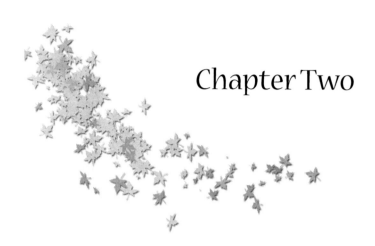

Chapter Two

What About Her Family?

I was overcome by . . . sorrow. PSALM 116:3

Unplanned pregnancies affect fathers-to-be as well as the parents and siblings of the mother- and father-to-be, their grandparents, aunts, uncles, cousins. . . . Even friends and co-workers or careers can be affected by an unplanned pregnancy. But it doesn't have to devastate lives or destroy relationships, even when it threatens to. For some families, the hardships and dilemmas brought by an unplanned pregnancy cause them to pull together and can even heal and strengthen relationships.

Sometimes those touched by an unplanned pregnancy just need someone to help them, to intervene. They need someone to hear them, to encourage and support them in good decisions. Here are the true stories of some families and women who found the help they needed.

29

Heartbroken Family

by Janne Strobel Collins

According to StateHealthFacts.org, percentages of legal abortions obtained in the United States by age group are as follows:

Up to 19 years old
17 %

20 ~ 30 years old
56 %

30 ~ 39 years old
23 %

40 years old and above
3 %

Age Unknown
1 % [1]

I had just swallowed the first bite of my lunch when the phone at the pregnancy care center rang. "My son's girlfriend is pregnant," a woman said. I could hear in her voice how distraught she was. "Her parents told her they won't allow her to have the baby. Can they do that?"

"The law says the woman has a right to choose. So it would be illegal to force someone to have an abortion," I told her. I tried to calm her, but I could hear loud voices in the background. "Could you encourage your son's girlfriend to come in for an appointment?"

"Her parents won't let her come near our son now," she said.

Those background voices grew louder. I could hear two men arguing, making loud comments. "Is everything okay where you are?" I asked.

"My husband is very upset," the woman said. "My son is trying to reassure him that he won't let anything happen to his girlfriend or their baby, but—"

"Can I talk to your son?" I asked. It took some coaxing, but finally I was able to talk with the son.

He was young, but he was adamant that he felt responsible for this life he had created. "I want this child with all my heart," he said. "I'm prepared to make sacrifices to look after my girlfriend and raise this child."

"Can you find a way to express that to your girlfriend and her parents?" I asked.

A strong voice continued in the background. This young man's father's negative comments made it very hard to counsel him over the phone.

"Dad," the son said, "you need to talk to this lady." He handed him the phone.

As I listened to the father, I could see that although this Dad was a Christian, he was having trouble trusting God with the outcome of this situation. As we spoke, he cried out, "*I failed my son!* I tried to teach him right. But I must have done something wrong." He blamed himself for his son's mistakes. We talked for a long time about his son and how sometimes children do things we wish they wouldn't, things we've taught them not to do. I tried to help him see how his son's willingness to be responsible for the baby was a sign that he had absorbed good teachings from his father. He calmed down and began to feel like there was hope again.

Before we hung up, I spoke with the mother again. "I just wanted to encourage you one last time to help this girl make an appointment with our pregnancy center," I said. "I suggest you *all* come in to talk—your family, her family. . . . " She agreed to contact the girl and her parents.

Later that day I received a call from the girlfriend. She made an appointment and both families came in for counseling. The counselor persuaded them to pull together, instead of apart, for the sake of their kids and the grandbaby. They left having decided against abortion and both families are now working together to plan a good life for this child.

It is wonderful when families pull together and work together for the good of the mom-to-be and the coming child, but it isn't always that way. Unlike the family Janne spoke with, Tina's family didn't pull together to help her. Tina's mother came from a strict Japanese culture. When Tina desperately needed her mother's help and support, her mother shunned her. Tina felt hopeless. Here is Tina's story as she told it to writer Sue Tornai.

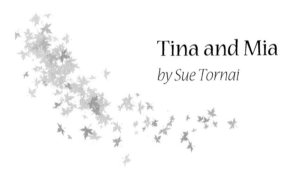

Tina and Mia

by Sue Tornai

Tina's family was never close. They didn't come around each other and they didn't talk with each other. Tina always tried to please her mother, but her mother's strong morals and Japanese culture made having a baby out of wedlock unacceptable. Tina was pregnant, and she brought shame to her home.

Tina's mother insisted she have an abortion. Under that insistence, Tina called several places that provide abortions, but she couldn't talk to anyone—each time she called either the office was not open or the counselor wasn't in.

"I was so scared of the vacuum procedure," Tina said. "I envisioned it tearing my baby apart. But Mom said the baby wasn't developed yet. I was ten weeks pregnant.

"I could only think of suicide," Tina said. "If I had to kill my baby, I might as well kill myself. I couldn't live with myself if I killed this life inside of me."

Long before her pregnancy, Tina was a self-mutilator—cutting herself, hurting herself when stressed. Scars lay across her arms in rows like the slats of a baby's crib.

32

"I hadn't cut myself for a long time," Tina said. But when she found out she was pregnant, Tina tightened her fist around a mirror until it broke. Her fingers found a shard, and she felt the temptation to cut again. Tina said, "I thought it would be okay since I wanted to kill myself anyway."

Depressed, lonely, and afraid, Tina desperately looked for someone who wasn't close to her family, someone she could talk to, someone who could help her.

Fortunately before she cut herself, she called Alternatives Pregnancy Resource Center in Sacramento, California. "She was distraught about having an abortion," said Kathy Hoover, a client advocate at the center. "I heard her cry for help. She wanted a lifeline."

The first time Tina came to the Center, she received the encouragement she longed for—someone told her she could keep her baby.

"When Tina left that day, I saw the weight she carried in with her had lifted from her shoulders," Kathy said. "Yet I knew she had to face her family with her decision."

"I lost everyone around me," Tina said. Her mom was still very unhappy about her pregnancy so when she began to show, Tina had to hide in her own house. When her mother had friends into their home, Tina had to stay out of sight. "It was hard to keep my baby," Tina says. "I kept telling my mom how I wished she would support me. She was all I had. She had always been my best friend. But now she distanced herself from me."

During Tina's second appointment with Kathy, she shared how she had been abandoned by her family and friends. "I was concerned whether she would continue her pregnancy," Kathy said. "Tina assured me she knew she had made the right decision."

The once-shy Tina started keeping her appointments with Kathy and with her doctor. She didn't just talk about doing things she had to do—she actually followed through. She stopped associating with the men who had abused her. When she felt sad, she didn't cut herself anymore. Instead, she talked

things out. She started eating right, and she chose to listen to happy music so she would be happy.

"When she saw a change in me, Mom started coming around," Tina said. "I think she saw how much I was trying to turn my life around. Sometimes I wonder if this pregnancy happened for a reason. My mom sees now how God used this pregnancy to improve my life."

Tina gave birth to a little girl. "Everything is about Mia now," Tina said. "Mia is the center of a family that does things together. My dad can't get away from her. He spoils her. He's always holding her. Mia's his baby girl.

"I wouldn't be here if it wasn't for you," Tina told Kathy at the pregnancy center. "I really connected with you. I could talk with you. I didn't feel I had to lie or shut you out. Right away you were helpful and supportive. You made me feel like I was right in my decision, and I thank God that I had Mia."

Tina knew she wanted to keep her child from the beginning, but it took a while for her family to come around and support her decision. At times it is just the reverse: the young mother doesn't know if she wants to carry the child while her family wants her to.

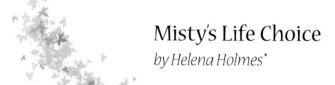

Misty's Life Choice

by Helena Holmes*

When I picked up the phone that morning, I heard my daughter, Rose*, say, "Mom? Misty* is pregnant." I could hear the sorrow in her voice.

"Are you sure?" I asked. Troubling emotions rushed over me. My granddaughter, Rose's fifteen-year-old daughter, is a smart, attractive, typical teenager.

"She did two pregnancy tests and they both showed positive," Rose said. "Her boyfriend wants her to get an abortion."

In the United States, more than six million women become pregnant annually

~ and ~
- *slightly fewer than two thirds result in live births;*

- *20% result in abortions;*

- *the remainder end in miscarriage.* [3]

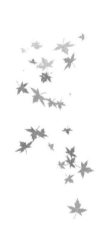

In 2002, an estimated 757,000 pregnancies among teenagers 15 to 19 years old resulted in: 425,000 live births, 215,000 induced abortions, and 117,000 fetal losses.

The overall teenage pregnancy rate was estimated at 76.4 pregnancies per 1,000 females aged 15–19 years~ Down 10% from 2000 (84.8 per 1,000), and 35% lower than the peak rate in 1990 (116.8 per 1,000).

The 2002 rate was an historic low for the nation. Rates for young teenagers declined relatively more than for older teenagers throughout this twelve-year period. [4]

As a volunteer at our local pregnancy center, I knew the critical influence a boyfriend could have in the decisions of a newly pregnant mother, especially a young mother. Rose was adamant about not wanting Misty to get an abortion, but she knew her daughter was in a fragile circumstance.

"Ask her if I can pick her up after school tomorrow," I said. "We can go to the pregnancy center and talk about this."

Rose quickly agreed. "I'll tell Misty," she said.

Besides volunteer counselors, our center has a nurse on staff and an ultrasound machine. When a mother is undecided about carrying her baby, the center offers her a free ultrasound so she can see the baby's image on screen.

When we arrived at the pregnancy center, Misty willingly talked with another volunteer counselor on staff. They did another pregnancy test to confirm she was pregnant. When the test showed positive, the counselor asked Misty if she would like to see the baby on the ultrasound. Misty emerged from the ultrasound room excited, telling me all about the baby. She had made the decision to carry her baby at that point.

The counselor referred Misty to a medical doctor and arranged to talk with her again in a few days. In future visits to the pregnancy center, the counselor talked with Misty about the possibility of placing her baby for adoption. Misty didn't want to do that. She wanted to parent her child, knowing it would be hard financially. Misty's boyfriend would not support her decision.

Our pregnancy center offers free parenting classes for young mothers, and Misty signed up. She received vouchers as a reward for attending all the classes, and she used them to purchase a changing table, clothes for her and for the baby, toys, blankets, and a several-month supply of diapers.

Misty faced some hard times, with some physical challenges during the pregnancy. Harder still was dealing with the rejection of her boyfriend. But a month after Misty turned sixteen, she gave birth to an eight-pound eleven-ounce dark-haired girl. She named her Mallary* and calls her Mally.*

Misty has no regrets. "Having Mallary was the best thing that happened to me," she said. "I was making bad choices and was headed for self-destruction. Mally helped me get my head in check."

Four-year-old Mallary is vivacious, independent, headstrong, healthy, and cute as a button. She is loved by all who know her, especially her parents, grandparents, and great-grandparents. What a delight and a blessing to have her in our lives. Our family is thankful for the support and help of the pregnancy center in our time of need.

When the staff at a pregnancy center pours their lives into helping others in unplanned pregnancies, it can be especially devastating to learn their own family is suddenly in that same situation. That's what happened to Helena and her family. That also happened to Lucy Neeley Adams's friend, Susan. Even with all her training as a volunteer at a pregnancy center, Susan struggled to deal with her daughter's news.*

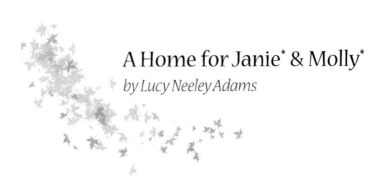

A Home for Janie* & Molly*

by Lucy Neeley Adams

I was a brand new, very frightened volunteer at the pregnancy center in Murfreesboro, Tennessee, so I asked Cliff, the center's director, if I could work the first few weeks at the front desk. I didn't tell him how frightened I was about counseling. I just knew I could at least answer the phones. But then I received the phone call I least expected.

"Oh Lucy, I'm so glad you're at the phone!" I recognized Susan's voice, a fellow counselor at the center. "I can't come back as a counselor," she cried. "Please tell Cliff I must resign."

"Susan," I said softly, "please calm down and tell me why you feel you must stop working here. And tell me why you can't come in to tell Cliff yourself."

"Lucy, my own daughter, Janie, is pregnant," Susan said. I knew her high-school-aged daughter. "How can I counsel others and urge them to abstain from premarital sex when I can't control my own daughter?!" Susan sobbed. "How can I help others find answers to life's questions when I have none of my own?" Susan paused to blow her nose. "And that's not even the worst of it, Lucy," Susan said barely above a whisper.

> **Black women are more than three times**
> **as likely as white women**
> **to have an abortion.**
>
> **Hispanic women are roughly two times**
> **as likely to have an abortion as white women.**[5]

"Tell me," I said gently.

"Janie is pregnant with a biracial baby!" Susan sobbed and sobbed over the phone.

I said, "Susan, listen to me. You have to come in to tell Cliff this news. He needs to hear it from you." She agreed and when she came in, I hugged her and cried with her. Later I watched Susan leave the place where she had loved to work.

In the following weeks, Janie came into the center for a pregnancy test and for counseling. By then I had progressed to that work and Janie became my client. Because I knew and loved Janie's whole family, she gladly counseled with me. I soon learned Janie was making her own plans to go to a maternity home.

"Usually a whole family is in on the decision of a maternity home," I told her. "Are you sure you want to do this?"

"I'm keeping my baby," she said. "My boyfriend said he will not marry me. And I heard he got another girl pregnant, too. I won't show my face at that high school again." I understood.

"Who will help you after the baby is born?" I asked.

"That's no problem," Janie said. "My family is so close and full of love. I'll come back home, of course."

After declining steadily from 1991–2005, birth rates for fifteen to nineteen-year-olds increased significantly between 2005 and 2006.

The overall teen birth rate increased 4% between 2005 and 2006, and another 1% between 2006 and 2007.

Preliminary birth data from 2008 show a 2% decrease from the 2007 teen birth rate, to slightly below the 2006 rate.

Underlying causes for the previous increase and subsequent decrease are not yet known, and it is unclear whether the rise will continue. Birth rates for other age groups also increased during this time.[6]

I felt a twinge. *Would it be that simple?* I wondered. *Does she know how her mother is struggling with her carrying a biracial child?*

Only a few days later, I was in the center early to meet with a new client. I thought this young girl's name sounded familiar. Her pregnancy test showed she was pregnant. When she wrote down the name of the father . . . that's when I knew. She was pregnant by the same boy as Janie. However, respecting confidentiality of all clients, I could say nothing to this girl, or to Janie, or to Susan.

Later that afternoon, I met with both Janie and Susan. The incident earlier that day prompted me to confirm to Janie and Susan that I felt in my heart Janie was making the right decision to go to a maternity home in another town. Together the three of us made plans to visit several homes. It was not my "job" to go with them, but this family was so close to me we all planned to go together.

But then Janie dropped the bombshell. "Mom doesn't want my baby," she said. "I won't be able to return home after the baby is born. Now we have to find me and my baby a place to live after she arrives."

Immediately Susan cried out, "Janie, this is a biracial baby! It needs an African American home."

"Mother," Janie said, "I have not told you yet, but I saw Dr. Sawyer last week." She patted her tummy. "This is not an 'it.' My baby is a girl. She will be precious, and you will love her dearly if you will just take us home."

I listened as they bickered back and forth. When they got up to leave, I quickly led them in a closing prayer, but the room was bulging with tension. I knew there would be many words between them as they returned home to Susan's husband and Janie's father, the grandfather-to-be. He was an outstanding lawyer in our town and had a quiet strength. I felt he would be a strong decision-maker in this confusion. Evidently he was because many good things began to unfold.

They were a loving Christian family and prayed about every move they made. They agreed upon which maternity home easily. They chose a home with a hospital nearby that would make it easy for them to get there quickly when the time came.

However, unbeknownst to Janie, I learned Susan had continued to make her own plans. She told me her story. Susan had been working to have her grandchild given for adoption. She had chosen an adoption agency. She had actually spoken to a counselor and was planning to choose a family to adopt her grandchild. The day came when Susan sat at the agency looking through picture books of parents who wanted to adopt babies. But Susan began to cry bitterly. Through her tears she prayed, "Oh God, look at all these beautiful people who long to be parents. When my husband and I were young, you blessed us with our dear daughter, Janie. Now do you want to bless us with her baby? Are we to be grandparents who will take Janie and her baby girl into our home?"

During the difficult months of Janie's pregnancy, Susan had memorized words from Psalm 37, and the opening words of that Psalm now came to her mind: "Do not fret." It seemed to Susan those words came directly from the voice of God. "Those words are written three times in the first eight verses of that Psalm," Susan told me. "I began to understand that if I did not fret, God would show the way . . . His way."

Susan told me she left that adoption agency with new determination to have peace as she prayed for God's will in her family. She knew this would be big news to her family, and the first person she had to tell was her husband.

The quietness of their empty house with Janie in the maternity home and the other children away at college had brought them closer together than ever. Susan loved and trusted her husband's decisions . . . on most things. But she had not trusted him about the adoption of their grandchild. Those thoughts had been hers alone. Now she had good news to share with him about her change of heart. She opened her Bible to read him those first eight verses of Psalm 37. Yes, there was that last phrase: "Do not fret—it only causes harm" (NKJV).

"Can we just not say anything to Janie about this for a while?" Susan asked her husband. "It could be that Janie will one day agree the best thing is to place this child for adoption. If that happens, we can all be at peace."

But that day never came. I talked with Susan shortly after the birth. Susan told me the biggest news of all: "I received this little baby girl, Molly, and Janie into our home." Susan said one of their other children was angry with that decision, but within weeks the whole family was in agreement. "We had a glorious springtime," Susan said. "It spoke of new life and new love. God had healed each of us in His way. Now I don't know how we could ever love a precious little one more than we do our Molly.

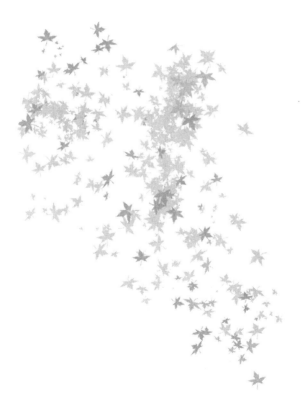

Resources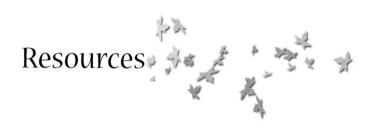

"Whatever help and options you need, search for them . . . because they are out there, waiting to be found.

 Pregnancy centers' trained counselors can help not only women in unplanned pregnancies, but also men and whole families. You can find a pregnancy center near you using the Resources listed at the end of Chapter 1.

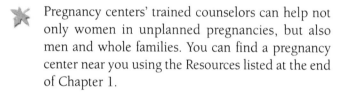 Book:
Mom, Dad, I'm Pregnant:
When Your Daughter or Son Faces
an Unplanned Pregnancy
by Jayne Schooler (NavPress, 2004).

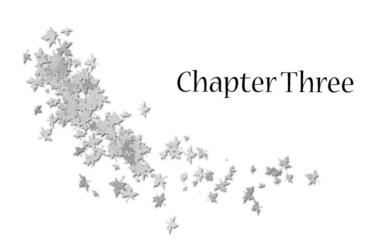

Chapter Three

When a Woman Considers Abortion

*The cords of death entangled me, the anguish
of the grave came upon me.*
PSALM 116:3

When a woman and a man find
themselves in an unplanned or unwanted
pregnancy, often the first option that comes to
mind is abortion. Women (and men) facing
unplanned or unwanted pregnancies consider
abortion for many reasons. But some want to
make other choices, and will, when given
hope, help, and other options.

In the following stories, we'll see these
women struggle with their decisions.

45

What Some May Call a Mistake

by Tina Brock

I'm the director of the Franklin Life Crisis Pregnancy Center in Carnesville, Georgia, and when I first saw our listing in the yellow pages, I was horrified. The phone company had mistakenly listed our center not only under "Abortion Alternatives" where it should have been, but also under "Abortion Services." Needless to say we started getting more calls inquiring about abortion.

I remember one young lady who came in for an appointment with one of our counselors. She had torn the "Abortion Services" page out of the yellow pages. After her appointment, she handed it to me on her way out the door and said, "I don't need this anymore."

Nine months later, she walked back in with a big smile on her face and a beautiful baby girl in her arms.
Because of that listing, we have seen women choose something other than abortion, and I know their lives are different because of it. All due to what some may call a mistake.

1% of all abortions occur because of rape or incest.

6% of abortions occur because of potential health problems regarding either the mother or child.

93% occur for "social reasons" (i.e. the child is unwanted or inconvenient). [1]

Her Soul Question

by Janne Strobel Collins

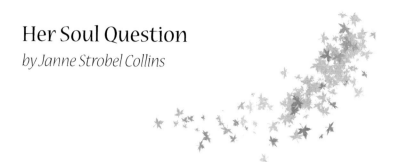

She was scared she was pregnant. She admitted she was a Christian who had "not been living right." Although she didn't like the thought of abortion, she would consider this option in order to "get out of the mess" she was in.

When she told the guy she was seeing she might be pregnant, she found out he didn't really love her. He swore "it" wasn't his and dumped her. She was devastated. Certain that her church family would also disown her if they found out about her lifestyle, she began avoiding church. She felt overwhelmed and alone. Abortion was looking more and more like a solution to her problem.

Then she asked me, "When would it be too late?"

"What do you mean 'too late'?" I asked.

"Too late for an abortion," she said. "I mean, when exactly does the soul enter the child?"

I had never been asked this question before. I explained to her that God clearly tells us in the Scriptures that He knew us before we were conceived in our mothers' wombs and that the soul is present from the moment of conception. "Before I formed you in the womb I knew you," God said through the prophet in Jeremiah 1:5. "Before you were born I set you apart."

I shared with her about the depth of God's love and care for us. "God has made a good plan for our lives," I said, "and if we will draw close to Him, He will work everything out for our good."

As we waited for her test results, she seemed very thoughtful. When the timer went off we saw that her test was negative. I took the opportunity to ask, "Would you like to get your life back on track with God?"

She wept. "Yes, I really would," she said. "I'm sick of living like this." We bowed our heads and prayed together. Then we talked about the steps to take to make this a lasting change, like reading the Bible daily and attending a good Bible-teaching church so we can know how God wants us to live, and then obeying what we learn. She left with a Bible and study materials in hand, and a new outlook. The smile on her face said it all.

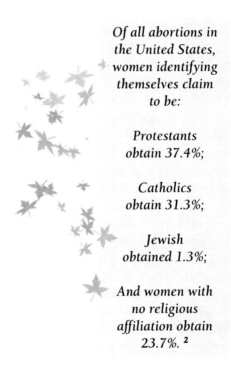

Of all abortions in the United States, women identifying themselves claim to be:

Protestants obtain 37.4%;

Catholics obtain 31.3%;

Jewish obtained 1.3%;

And women with no religious affiliation obtain 23.7%. [2]

Sometimes the staff at a pregnancy center never discovers what decision a client ultimately makes. But sometimes they do. Here are two stories from people who, at least for a time, truly didn't know how the story ended.

God Will Forgive Me

*by Marcia Samuels**
as told to Dianne E. Butts

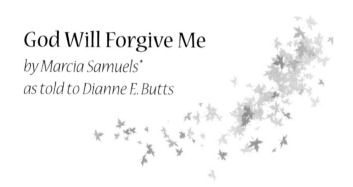

I was working in a small town pregnancy center when a young woman came in. She already knew she was pregnant. "I've been accepted into the military," she said. "I can't go into the military pregnant."

She told me she'd already had one abortion. She didn't want to have another; the first had caused her such pain. Still, her dilemma was that she could not remain pregnant and also join the military.

"I'm a Christian," she said. "I know God will forgive me."
Of all abortions in the United States, women identifying themselves as:

"If you believe you will need God's forgiveness, then you also believe abortion is wrong," I told her. "God loves each of His children and He will forgive us for our sins, but there are still consequences for doing what is wrong. His forgiveness doesn't make the consequences go away."

She left the pregnancy center that day and I never heard from her again.

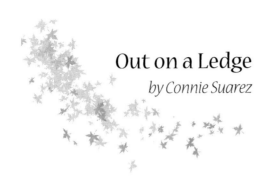

Out on a Ledge

by Connie Suarez

I work as a counselor in a small town pregnancy center. Anita* walked in wanting a free pregnancy test. While I waited with her for the results, I asked her, "What are your plans if you're pregnant?"

"I just can't be pregnant," Anita said. Tears welled in her eyes.

"Last night, my husband Jake* left me. I've got to have back surgery, so I called the doctor's office and told them I might be pregnant. The nurse said that wouldn't be good."

As Anita poured out the heartbreak of her crumbling marriage and difficult life, I listened.

"It would help if I could talk to my mother right now," Anita continued, "but she's been sick and I hate to burden her. I have to be strong for my other children. I haven't yet told them Jake left. What am I going to do?"

I tried hard to follow what I'd learned in counselor training: it wasn't my responsibility to make decisions for Anita. I could support her, offer her information and options, but Anita had to make her own choices about what to do.

We looked at the pregnancy test together. Two lines. Anita looked back and forth between the two lines and the results table on the empty box as if hoping one line might disappear. Finally, in a ragged voice, she said, "Positive. It's positive." She began to cry. My eyes were welling with tears for her.

I left Anita for a few minutes and went to the rack where our pregnancy center keeps a myriad of brochures and pamphlets. I picked out two. It seemed so little, but I gave Anita the brochure titled, "Before You Decide." I showed her the pages that talked about abortion procedures and risks. Anita spent a long time looking at the pages showing the development of a fetus over the months of pregnancy. Then I gave her a small card that said, "We're Glad You Came." It contained Bible verses, but I didn't get a chance to share them with Anita.

Anita left. I felt overwhelmed with grief and guilt. I tried to think of what I could have said or done differently. What more could I have done to help Anita?

My coworkers knew those same feelings all too well. So we talked. And we prayed for Anita. Even so, I felt sure abortion would be Anita's choice. I know many women who regret their choice to abort. I couldn't believe that was really a great option for Anita, but it was just so hard for me to see how she might choose anything other than abortion.

After our talk and prayer, I felt encouraged and hopeful. We ended our day at the center, turning off the equipment and switching the phone to forward to the twenty-four hour help line volunteer. When we walked out the door and pulled it shut behind us, we saw the brochures. Both pieces of literature I had given Anita lay out on a brick ledge near the door. "She didn't even take them with her," I said.

I continued to pray for Anita with my coworkers at the pregnancy center, but we didn't hear anything more from her. Days and weeks passed. Weeks turned into months.

One day a woman with a four-month-old baby came in for some baby clothes. She picked out what she needed then left.

"Didn't she seem familiar?" I asked my coworkers. It took some discussion before we figured it out. It had been more than a year since I had met Anita and she had left the brochures out on the ledge, but that was Anita. And that was her baby.

Resources

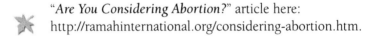

 Women have more options than abortion or abortion clinics. Pregnancy centers train counselors to help a woman know all the resources available to her and to think through all her options. Find a pregnancy center near you at http://www.optionline.org/.

"Are You Considering Abortion?" article here:
http://ramahinternational.org/considering-abortion.htm.

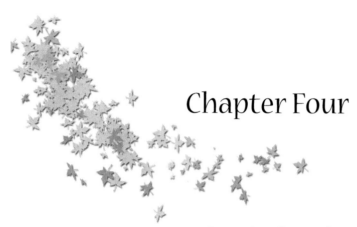

Chapter Four

Learning from Those
Who Have Experienced Abortion

Then I called on the name of the LORD:
O LORD, save me!" . . . For you, O LORD,
have delivered my soul from death, my eyes from tears,
my feet from stumbling, that I may walk before the LORD
in the land of the living . . . You have freed me from my chains.

PSALM 116:4, 8–9, 16

When a woman has an abortion that's the end of it. That's the end of the pregnancy. The baby. The problem. The issue. It's over. Right?

Think again.

Here, several women who have experienced abortion share their stories. Sharing their story wasn't easy for any of them, but they hope that knowing what they experienced will help you make your decision, inspire you, help you heal, or know that you are not alone.

They'll answer your questions. Why did she choose abortion? How did it affect her? Were there any lingering aftereffects? If yes, how did she deal with them?

Where is she now with all of it? Has she recovered? What has she learned, and what is she doing with all she has learned?

Whether two years ago or twenty, whether she has had one abortion or several, here is her story.

It's Never Over

by Tina Brock

Of U. S. women obtaining abortions, 18% are teenagers. Of those 11% are 18-19 years old;

6% are 15-17 years old;

0.4% are under age 15 [1]

I had just graduated from high school and turned eighteen when I learned I was pregnant. Most of my family and friends advised me not to have the baby. I thought my only option was abortion. I had no facts about abortion. No one, including me, including my family and friends, knew the effects an abortion would have on my life.

I was scared about becoming pregnant at this time in my life. I was riding an emotional roller coaster. I cried day after day because I wasn't sure what to do.

About a month after my eighteenth birthday, I found myself lying on an abortionist's table in Atlanta, Georgia.

The nurse held my hand and told me it would be over soon, but that was a lie. My abortion is never over.

In the following years, I suffered depression, anxiety attacks, and nightmares. Every year in August I would think about how old my baby would be.

A few years ago, I attended an abortion recovery Bible study at the crisis pregnancy center where I was volunteering. I found myself forgiven by God and set free from the shame, guilt, and anguish of my abortion experience. I only wish there had been a crisis pregnancy center there for me when I needed one, a center that would have shared with me the truth about abortion and all of my options.

I worked at the pregnancy center in Jackson County for two years. Then I went back to my hometown where I had lived when I needed a pregnancy center nearly nineteen years earlier. I opened Franklin Life Crisis Pregnancy Center in Carnesville, Georgia. I'm here to help women. I give them the facts about abortion that I was never told so they don't have to go through what I went through.

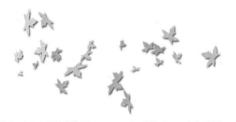

Professional counselors recognize common reactions, together called "Post-Abortion Syndrome," some women experience after abortion.

They include: anxiety, emotional numbing, difficulty recalling the event, guilt, grief, depression, anger, aggressive behavior, flashbacks, nightmares, anniversary reactions, alcohol abuse, drug abuse, and suicidal thoughts.[2]

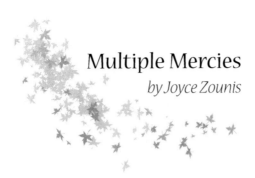

Multiple Mercies
by Joyce Zounis

"Don't tell *anyone* of this," Mother whispered.

It was 1977 and I was fifteen when we walked into the abortion facility. I felt aggravated that I had to be there. I was missing cheerleading practice, completely disconnected from what was about to happen. My emotions had shut down long ago . . .

When I was six years old, we loaded up the family station wagon and headed south to visit my cousins in the country. When we arrived, I saw cornstalks taller than anything Mom had ever planted in our suburban backyard.

My younger cousin called, "C'mon, Joyce!" and ran into the cornfield. I ran in after him. "C'mon slowpoke!" he hollered. I fought my way through the corn to catch up. When I did . . . he touched me where he should not have touched me. Frightened, I sensed this was very, very bad, but I was too afraid to tell anyone, especially my strict military father. So the sexual abuse continued for several summers. No one knew this secret.

While my father was away serving in the military, Sunday mornings Mother would polish us up and off we'd go to church. I loved being there and learning about Jesus. I was eight years old when I proclaimed Jesus as my Savior. But I felt shame from the shadows of the cornfield. The next year at a church sleepover, I learned about purity and I finally knew what I was not.

When I became a teenager, those sexual violations turned into invitations. Well, I was already not "pure," right? I also began smoking pot and loved how it helped me escape the awful feelings I felt inside.

Then in 1977, I knew I was pregnant. I left my mom a note under her pillow. "We will never speak of this again," she whispered as we walked through the door. Another secret. But the waiting room was filled with girls and to my mom's dismay, we saw someone we knew. I just wanted it over so life could go back to normal.

The counselor told me it would be quick. I tuned out. It was a warm September day, but I remember feeling ice cold. I saw the tube fill with blood and tissue as the vacuum removed my first child. I was an empty shell of a mother.

Life did not go back to normal. I made the honor roll, performed on the cheerleading squad, and was elected homecoming queen. But inside I felt disconnected and empty.

My junior year I was sixteen and pregnant again. I told my boyfriend not to worry, that I would take care of it. We dated for five years, but our future marriage died the day I lay down on that abortion table.

After college I married another man. I had two abortions with him prior to our marriage and two during the marriage. I believed this was unconditional love, and I was willing to do anything to keep him in my life. But he had an adulterous relationship and we divorced.

47% of all abortions are performed on women who have had at least one previous abortion.[3]

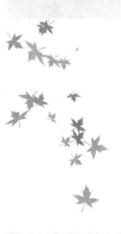

Of all abortions

Never-married women obtain 64.4%

Married women obtain 18.4%

Divorced women obtain 9.4%.[4]

I rebounded into another relationship and a year later I was pregnant. "I'm not going to have an abortion this time," I told myself. "I can't. I won't." I gave birth to my first living child, a beautiful boy. But while I delivered him, his father was in the arms of another woman.

It took me three months to let go of that relationship, and on the very day I did I met Ted Zounis. He loved me and my baby boy, and we were married five-and-a-half weeks later. Ted adopted my son and we renamed him Costa. Finally I had a real family.

Costa wrapped his tiny fingers around mine, and secretly my stomach churned at the thought of the babies I had aborted. Hot tears filled my eyes often, but never fell. Grief was followed closely by guilt and shame, but fear kept me from laying bare my secrets. No one, not even my husband, knew the truth.

Ted and I were excited to learn I was pregnant, however a difficult pregnancy lay ahead of me and Ted was often away serving in the military. I decided abortion was the solution. Ted was completely against it, but several weeks later he went with me to the abortion facility.

Eleven years had passed since my first abortion and here I was having my seventh at the very same facility. I pushed back the thoughts and feelings until the sound of the vacuum brought a flood of memories. I started crying. The doctor, with splattered blood on his gown, seemed indignant. Ted and I left that place and our child behind. When we arrived home, Ted went across the street and found solace in drugs. Ted felt the impact of that day for years.

Soon my job with a national hotel chain moved us to southern Florida. I thought I was pregnant, pulled out the yellow pages, and called a local facility for a free pregnancy test. I thought I had called an abortion facility. But when I arrived I was shocked to learn I had unknowingly called the Boca Raton Tender Loving Care (TLC) Pregnancy Center (now called First Care). TLC helped women and men with pregnancy-related concerns. I didn't even know places like this existed.

My pregnancy test, however, was inconclusive. We set another appointment for two weeks later. When I returned for another test, it was positive. The woman at the TLC Pregnancy Center asked if she could give me a hug. She celebrated. I was completely amazed. TLC offered to help Ted and me as we faced the challenge of having a second child with little income. That was new! I gave birth to our daughter, Melina.

Even though Ted and I both knew the Lord Jesus since childhood, we weren't living like Christians. Drugs were prevalent in our home. We never gave church a second thought. When Costa mimicked us smoking marijuana in public, we finally decided we needed to make some changes in our lives and our marriage. We'd been given a business card for a local church, and so we attended church together for the first time.

I can't remember a time I felt so enveloped by God's love. The faith of the little girl I used to be filled my heart once again. I always believed myself to be a Christian, but it had been easier to turn my back on Christ than to confront the reality of my actions.

We attended church weekly and soon Pastor Bob began to tell the congregation about an event called Life Chain on the first Sunday in October. My secret past haunted me, yet I was compelled to participate in the event. I stood with thousands of

Christians along a street for one hour of prayer. Though surrounded by Christians, I felt alone and isolated. The sign I held read "*Abortion Kills Children.*" It felt like fire in my hands.

Ted and I now had three children and only a few weeks later Ted took them out for a treat leaving me for a rare moment alone in a quiet house. I turned on Christian radio for the first time.

The guest on the radio show that day was Carol Everett, a former abortion facility operator. She shared how she had been indirectly involved with over 35,000 abortions—including her own.[6] Yet she called herself an ambassador of Jesus Christ by His mercy and grace. She told her story of God's forgiveness and healing of her past.

My big hang-up was my number. I'd had seven abortions. Right then in my heart and mind I heard God say, "Joyce, if I can forgive her with 35,000 abortions, I can forgive you." Tears I'd held back for years flowed freely from the hidden places in my heart. I finally got honest with God. All He had ever wanted was for me to tell Him the truth and ask for forgiveness. He had always loved me. He had never left me.

Later that year I thought I was pregnant again and so I visited TLC again. This time my pregnancy symptoms turned out to be false, but one of the ladies who worked there, Evelyn,* said, "Joyce, would you consider volunteering here at TLC? You have so much to offer other women with similar experiences."

"I . . . I don't know," I stammered. The next week I called Evelyn and asked, "Does the offer still stand?"

The following day Evelyn gave me a tour of the pregnancy center. She explained that every volunteer lay counselor fills out an application and, if they have experienced abortion, they are required to participate in the center's abortion recovery program. "It's called Post-Abortion Counseling and Education (PACE)," Evelyn explained. "It's a recovery Bible study."

I agreed to participate in PACE and filled out the application, although I lied about how many abortions I'd had. If they knew the truth, I feared they'd bounce me right out the door. PACE was a challenging and intimate time. I was able to embrace the process of grieving over my abortions, and was given the sure hope of being reunited with my babies in heaven. My experience with God's forgiveness and peace deepened, filling me with a joy I'd desperately needed since the past days of the cornfield.

Seven abortions and not once was I told the physical risks I could suffer because of abortion, which include a possibly increased chance of breast cancer, ovarian cysts, and placenta previa.

"If a woman gives birth before 32 weeks, or has an induced abortion, she will have an increased risk of breast cancer . . ." [7]

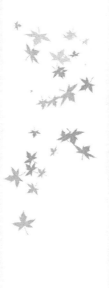

"Having several abortions using dilation and curettage (D&C) may create enough scar tissue to reduce a woman's ability to become pregnant and increases the risk of pregnancy complications, including ectopic pregnancy, miscarriage, and placenta previa." [8]

"Placenta previa is a placenta that has grown low in the uterus, partially or fully over the opening to the birth canal (cervix). Placenta previa can be dangerous during labor and delivery, when it is most likely to cause severe placental bleeding that can be life-threatening to the mother or fetus." [9]

63

A little over half (52%) of women obtaining abortions in the
U.S. are younger than 25 years old:

Teenagers obtain 20%
(with girls under 15 accounting for 1.2%);

Women 20 to 24 obtain 32%. [10]

During my most recent pregnancy, I developed placenta previa, a condition in which the placenta grows partially or completely over the opening of the birth canal and can cause extensive bleeding. During delivery, I lost all but two pints of blood and doctors had to perform a partial hysterectomy to stop the bleeding and save my life. I won't be able to have any more children.

Unfortunately, my marriage with Ted didn't last; he filed for divorce in February 2008. I am now the mother of twelve, with five living children: Costa, Melina, Niko, Teddy, and Mica.

Whether a woman has had many abortions or one, she may struggle afterwards. Where can she go for help? Who would understand? In the remaining stories in this chapter, you'll see where women found the help their hearts and souls longed for.

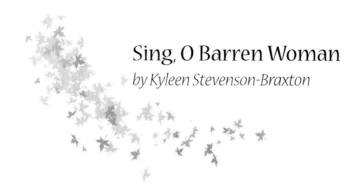

Sing, O Barren Woman

by Kyleen Stevenson-Braxton

I shifted uncomfortably in the leather chair waiting for the doctor. In front of me a massive cherrywood desk that dominated the room dwarfed the thin file lying in the center of it. It was my patient record sitting there, unmoving, holding essential information about my life.

The doctor entered, sat down, and opened the file. He lifted his eyes slowly. With a heavy sigh he said to me, "I was stunned by the results of your biopsy."

In the next moments, I learned I had stage IV cervical cancer. My life stopped. Because of the advanced stage of my cancer, the only treatment recommended was a hysterectomy.

I was twenty-eight years old, a newlywed, and facing barrenness.

Following my diagnosis and surgery, I struggled with fear, anger, and depression. I believed I was being punished for having had an abortion when I was nineteen.

Like so many others in my situation, I saw an abortion as a solution to a pregnancy that would have prevented me from finishing college and sent me back home in shame after my freshman year, a scenario I just couldn't imagine. Almost ten years later, I couldn't quite shake the feeling that I was getting what I deserved. I had squandered the first life God had placed in my care, and now that I was ready to begin having a family, who was I to expect another chance? It felt like justice.

All those years between my abortion and my cancer diagnosis, I lived in denial. I told myself it was just a blob of tissue and not a human being. I told myself I was making the best decision for my future. And most importantly, I told myself that God would forgive me.

I kept my secret hidden. I became incredibly driven to succeed in college. I think I needed to prove to myself that I had made the right choice. Getting my education became my rationalization and feminism became my excuse because it was *my* body. But that day in my doctor's office, God began to chip away at my carefully thought-out excuses.

Losing my ability to have children of my own caused me to confront my past. As everything I had chosen to believe about my choice came crashing down around me, it brought me to my knees. I beheld my sin through God's eyes: abortion takes a life and not a lump of cells. I was devastated.

But it was the beginning of my healing.

Over the next four years God began to deal with my wounded heart. He led me to Care Net Pregnancy and Resource Clinic of Casper, Wyoming, where I received post-abortion counseling and healing through the help of a Bible study written for post-abortive women called *Forgiven and Set Free*. I was shocked to learn about post-abortion stress syndrome and the health risks of abortion. I felt angry that I had not been given this information when I was making my choice. I recognized myself in the symptoms of post-abortion stress.

I realized that while I had accepted God's forgiveness and had forgiven myself, I had not yet begun to see my child as a real person—a child that needed to be grieved. I had been stuck in the grieving process, unable to move beyond depression and detachment into acceptance.

It seemed impossible to grieve a child that was not tangible to me. I sensed that I needed to ask God for a name for that child. So one day I sat down with pen and paper and prayed. Almost immediately the name "Holly Maria" came to my mind.

And so I began a letter to my child.

"Dear Holly . . ."

Through streaming tears I wrote to her about how sorry I was and about how deeply I missed her. I looked up the meaning of her names and learned that "Holly" means "pure spirit" and "Maria" means "living fragrance."

When I discovered her middle name comes from myrrh, the fragrance offered in worship to Jesus at His birth by the wise men, I imagined her as a worshipper dancing before the throne of God. Even now my eyes fill with tears as I recall that precious time and as I remember my sweet daughter.

It was God's plan to restore me. And in the process He gave me a passion for post-abortion ministry. I didn't count on being diagnosed with cancer, or being barren, or that someday my husband and I would be called to the healing ministry that is a crisis pregnancy center. But what I *really* didn't count on was God's mercy and restoration, and the joy that it brings.

On October 12, 2004, our adopted baby daughter was born. We asked God for a name, and He gave us "Maria." In addition to "living fragrance," the name also means "bitter waters" and comes from the story of the bitter waters of Marah in Exodus 15:22–25 in the Old Testament. Just as God made the waters sweet so His people could drink, He made my bitter waters sweet. And now, nearly twenty years later, my heart sings with the fruitfulness of two adopted children so that the words of Isaiah 54:1 ring in my ears: "'Sing, O barren woman, you who never bore a child; burst into song, shout for joy, you who were never in labor; because more are the children of the desolate woman than of her who has a husband,' says the LORD."

Psalm 71:20 and 23 says, "Though you have made me see troubles, many and bitter, you will restore my life again. . . . My lips will shout for joy when I sing praise to you." When I hold each of my two precious children in my arms, I sing praises to God in my heart . . . for His mercy, for His forgiveness, for His great kindness. And for unspeakable joy!

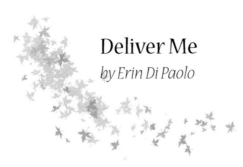

Deliver Me

by Erin Di Paolo

I was twenty-one years old, pregnant, and devastated. This couldn't be happening. I never dreamed I'd be in this position. Afraid, desperate, and alone, I made the only choice I thought I had.

As soon as I could, I made an appointment, went to a clinic, and did something I never thought I was capable of. I took the life of my own child, fully aware that's what I was doing. But I was not aware of the consequences my action would bring.

When I think of the shame of it all, it makes my heart sick. I lived with my parents, and they had no idea I was pregnant. The secrecy of my pregnancy and abortion brought me incredible guilt and shame. I became depressed and isolated myself even from my fiancé. Our relationship spiraled downward and never recovered. I partially blamed him, yet I knew there was no one to blame but myself.

Within days after my relationship with the baby's father ended, God brought me into a relationship with His Son, Jesus Christ. He delivered me from sin to salvation. But in areas of my living and thinking, He still had some delivering to do.

In an effort to justify my decision, I became even more outspoken on a woman's right to choose. The pain of the abortion remained, but I pushed it aside. I had not truly received God's forgiveness for this sin, and I had not forgiven myself. So even after I became a Christian, I remained pro-choice. I continued to live in denial.

But God would not leave me there.

As a new Christian, I became a devoted listener to Chuck

68

Swindoll's radio program, *Insight for Living*. Every month I would give a donation and request the book offer for that month. It was less than a year after I became a Christian when, much to my dismay, one month I received a different book than what I had requested. I received Chuck Swindoll's book *Sanctity of Life: The Inescapable Issue*. Was this a joke? I wondered why the ministry would send me *this* book by mistake. Why could I not escape this issue? I hadn't ordered it. I didn't *want* it! But God was not joking.

I determined I would never read that book. But, of course, once I said "never," I'm sure God just sat back and laughed. Hadn't He heard the word never from me before?

A short time passed before I picked up that book, and then I couldn't put it down. It was a wonderful book! I thought it would bring condemnation, but instead it brought healing. I remember it like it was yesterday. It was as if Christ Himself reached down from heaven, put His arms around me and said, "I died for *all* your sins. I love you."

I sobbed and sobbed. As I did, I felt this sweet sense of peace wash over me. I had been forgiven the sin I thought was unforgivable. In the New Testament, Romans 8:1 says, "There is now no condemnation for those who are in Christ Jesus." I genuinely understand what that verse means and I rejoice in the truth of it, for surely if there was a sin that would condemn me to hell it would be this one. But God says otherwise.

I told God I would do whatever He wanted me to do in the pro-life arena. Fifteen years ago I volunteered at a crisis pregnancy center in Denver, Colorado. This center ministers to women and men in crisis pregnancies and who are suffering the aftermath of abortion.

22% of all pregnancies in America
(excluding miscarriages)
end in abortion. [11]

Several years ago I attended a Christian post-abortion support group offered by the pregnancy center. I really didn't think I needed it, but I decided to go to minister to other women who needed to deal with their issues. I didn't think I had any issues left to deal with. But going through that group opened my eyes to pain and anger I didn't realize I had. It truly set me free! Participating in the group enabled me to also help many other women who were still in bondage, refusing to be set free, or not even knowing how to go about it.

We held a memorial service for our babies, complete with a pastor, Scripture reading, and music. We named our babies. Their names were read out loud—one by one. It was a beautiful tribute to the lives of our babies and sweet closure for all of us who grieved our losses.

It was awesome to witness each woman work through the grieving process and accept God's forgiveness while at the same time forgiving herself. Sometimes the hardest obstacle post-abortive women face is forgiving themselves, yet not doing so cheapens God's grace. If He forgives us, how can we possibly think we can't forgive ourselves?

If it had not been for my experience with that Denver pregnancy center, I do not know where I would be today. I'm grateful to God I don't have to find out. My abortion was many years ago, and I still grieve it. However I now know true forgiveness, and I know I will one day see my baby in heaven.

Living Well

by Ann Eppard

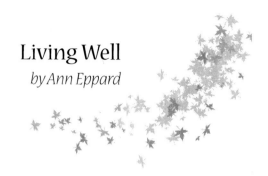

I picked up the phone. I set it down. I picked it up again. Finally, I dialed.

A woman answered. "Living Well Medical Clinic. This is Terry."

"Uh . . . hi," I stammered. "I want to volunteer at your clinic, but, I"—I felt God nudging me to go ahead—"but I've had an abortion."

"You know, many of our volunteers have had abortions," Terry said.

"They have?" I asked.

"Yes, and we offer a post-abortion Bible study."

A post-abortion Bible study? I thought. Unexpected words.

"In fact, one starts tomorrow night. Can you come in to register?"

God knew He would have to throw me into this.

My eleven-month old daughter napped and my boys played in the yard. "I think I can find a sitter," I told her. "Let me see what I can do." I got directions to the clinic and got my neighbor to watch the kids.

Thoughts rushed through my head as I drove. How did this happen? I was hoping to volunteer, to help someone else in crisis. *My repayment of sorts*, I thought. *My atonement.* But God, knowing my years of shame and guilt, knew I could never help another young pregnant woman until I worked through the scars of my own abortion.

I walked up the steps, not knowing what to expect. The sign on the door read "Living Well." The office looked like a doctor's: receptionist, magazines, lamp. My mind flashed back to that place where my abortion took place. A familiar twinge of guilt hit me in the gut.

Terry led me to an office and began to tell me about PACE. "Post-Abortion Counseling and Education meets every other week for twelve sessions," Terry said. "It's confidential."

My mind flashed back to that dark night just a few weeks ago, when in a fit of desperation and despair, I dropped to my knees and cried out to God, *Help me!*

Now God was reaching down from heaven with help. After twelve years, I was speaking with another Christian about my abortion. I felt shame, yes. But judgment? No. Guilt? Yes. Gentleness. *Yes!*

For twelve years I had lived in fear. *What if someone knew the real me? What would they think?* I had imagined picketers outside abortion clinics carrying signs: "Choose *Life!*" "Abortion *Kills.*" Those Christian soldiers angered and haunted me. I was a Christian at the time of my abortion. *What would you have done in my situation?!* I shouted back silently.

Terry handed me the book we would study in the group. I flipped through it and agreed to attend.

That was March of 1993. Almost exactly twelve years earlier, I was sixteen and pregnant. My high-school sweetheart, Rik, was the father. After the abortion we stayed together, broke up in college, then got back together after he became a Christian. We married after he graduated from college in '85, and we had Justin in '87. Rik joined the Marine Corps in 1989. Connor was born in 1990 and Erika in '92. In early 1993, I thought, *We have three beautiful children. I have all I ever wanted. So why am I so unhappy?*

Rik and I had decided together to have no more babies. That's when the reality of our aborted child suddenly haunted me. I told people I had three children, but the truth was I had four. It was as if a dark canopy kept the sun from shining through. I was angry or sad all the time. I shook my finger in Justin's little face. I yelled. I cried. It was always gray outside. Dingy. Dark. That's when I had cried out to God, *Help me!*

That evening, I told Rik about the PACE study. A Marine Corps pilot, he was preoccupied, focused on preparing for a six-month deployment. He didn't say much. For me, though, the darkness had to be dealt with.

When I walked into that support group, I didn't think there would be other Christian women who'd had abortions. I truly thought I was the only one. But I was not.

As the twelve weeks of PACE rolled into months, I walked through many emotions and memories. I had bitterness buried deep in my heart toward my husband, my parents, my in-laws, and the doctor who performed the abortion. My unforgiving heart festered with anger and pain, and had caused the depression that now haunted me. All that had to be dealt with. But first I had to forgive myself.

I believed my sin of abortion was a bigger sin than any other I had committed. Through the study, I learned that sin is sin. *All* of my sins needed the loving forgiveness of the Father. Jesus, through His loving sacrifice on the cross, had died for every one of my sins. Until then *grace, forgiveness,* and *hope* were words

Eighteen percent of all abortions are performed on women who identify themselves as "Born-again /Evangelical." [12]

Nearly eight in ten U.S. women obtaining an abortion report a religious affiliation:

43% report they are Protestant,

27% report they are Catholic,

8% report they are another religion. [13]

meant for other Christians. But today, they are for me. What were once just Bible verses became living words to heal and help me.

Through writing in a journal, reading God's Word, and praying, slowly I was able to forgive the people who had been involved in my abortion. And I grieved for the child who died in my selfish act on May 14, 1981. I named her Sarah. I looked at my other three children in a new light. I loved them even more, appreciating their little hugs.

Finally the darkness lifted and I began to see the sky.

I still grieve each December when Sarah would have been born. Each Easter I remember the anniversary of my abortion. Mother's Day brings joy for my children and sadness for my child who I aborted. But even so, because of that group at Living Well Medical Clinic and that wonderful Bible study, I truly am living well.

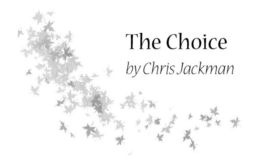

The Choice

by Chris Jackman

I was twenty-two, recovering from a failed marriage, and a single mom of a two-year-old son when I found myself in an unplanned pregnancy. Out of fear and self-protection, I chose abortion. My boyfriend drove me to the clinic.

Lying on the cold table, listening to the sound of the suction machine, I felt my spirit grow numb. The moment I walked out of that abortion clinic, I knew I would never be the same.

Regret and unresolved grief soon led to self-destructive behaviors and relationships. I could not live with the knowledge of what I had done: I had taken the life of my own child. How could I, as a woman, have done that? I loathed myself and tried to bury my abortion experience with the short-term pain management of denial, but it colored my life . . . my thoughts . . . my actions. Suicidal depressions came over me, and I often found myself in the bathroom with a razor poised at my wrist trying to work up the courage to end my torment. I couldn't talk about the abortion with anyone. I was too ashamed to admit it. I hid for years.

One awful night, I couldn't run from it any longer. I cried out to God, pleading for His forgiveness. A supernatural wave of peace washed over me, and I knew I was completely forgiven.

Sometime later I heard of an abortion recovery support group and Bible study. I didn't think I needed the group because I knew God had forgiven me. But I had unfinished business. If I was truly okay about it, why couldn't I talk to anyone about it? I joined the group and realized I hadn't grieved the loss of my child. The support group allowed me to grieve. The ten-week class ended with a memorial service for the participants' babies and I found a sense of closure and, amazingly, freedom!

A few years passed. Late one night in the spring of 1998, a song came over the radio. Kathy Troccoli's "A Baby's Prayer" brought me to my knees weeping. That song is a compassionate message of grace and forgiveness for a mother who had aborted her child. I

Women suffering

Post-Abortion

Syndrome may

experience:

- alcohol abuse

- drug abuse

- and may even

attempt suicide [14]

75

felt the tears of heaven. I again cried out to God, *Lord, please, however, whatever You want me to do to help make a difference, use me.*

Only a few days later, I talked with a Christian bookstore owner about those wounded by abortion. "Chris, you're a songwriter," he said. "Why don't you make your next CD project about abortion recovery?"

Why hadn't I thought of that? I walked out the door saying, *Okay, Lord. If this is it, give me the songs, the people, the money needed to make it happen.* I got everything I asked for and more.

In the summer of '98 I spent weekends cloistered in a secluded log cabin praying and writing songs for my project, *The Choice*. Reliving my abortion experience and recovery was emotionally exhausting. As I recounted the abortion and subsequent years of pain, each song brought me to my knees in tears. Then, in tears of joy I rediscovered the astounding grace, mercy, and love of Christ for me.

I brought friend and fellow songwriter Cordell Langeland aboard as producer and musical cowriter. A wonderful team of people helped to make *The Choice* CD a reality. *The Choice* is a ten-song musical CD designed to reach out to hurting post-abortive women and men with the mercy, grace, and restoration of Jesus Christ.

Pregnancy centers, abortion recovery ministries, churches, and individuals throughout the United States have used *The Choice* CD. My desire is to educate the church and society of the reality of post-abortion trauma and its devastating affects.

It's estimated that 43% of all women will experience at least one abortion by age forty-five. That breaks my heart. I know many women and men involved in abortion will go through what I did. I would spare them that if I could.

An estimated 43% of all women will have at least one abortion by the time they are 45 years old. [15]

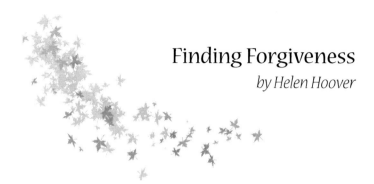

Finding Forgiveness

by Helen Hoover

"You can't understand," Claire* told me emphatically. "You haven't done all the things I've done." Claire was a middle-aged lady whose life was in shambles because of the bad choices she'd made in her younger years. Now she was divorced, living on welfare, in poor health, and depressed. The director of our center, Life Choices in Joplin, Missouri, had encouraged Claire to take the post-abortion class I led as part of my volunteer service to the center.

"You're right," I told her. "I've never had an abortion. I've never committed adultery. I never took drugs or smoked or drank liquor. But I have been critical, greedy, prideful, judgmental, and have lied to others. That's just a few of my sins."

Claire wanted help and therefore had agreed to come to the meetings. She was a willing participant, did her homework, and shared her life. But when we came to the lesson on God's forgiveness, the immensity of her sins stymied her. She struggled with the concept that God's forgiveness applied to her.

"Forgiveness from God is not based upon what sin we've committed," I explained. "Our forgiveness is based upon Jesus' death on the cross."

Claire's face began to show understanding. We discussed how Christ's death on the cross paid the death penalty for our sins and applied to each one of us who would accept His sacrifice on our behalf, as Claire had already done. The despicable things we had indulged in did not negate His forgiveness available to us.

With time, talking, and the study's lessons, Claire came to understand and accept God's forgiveness for her. Within a few months, she started taking classes to apply for a position at a hospital. She gradually backed off the medication for depression and started leading a productive life. As leader of the group, I'm constantly delighted to see God work in the participant's lives.

Mildred* came to class at the invitation of a friend, who was another participant. She had gone to a professional counselor to deal with the emotional hang-over of three abortions. The last night of our class she told me, "That counselor tried to help me, but he didn't tell me about God's forgiveness. I thought I would always be unforgiven for the abortions." Her face beamed as she told us how thankful she was for God's forgiveness.

At Life Choices, we also offer group studies for married couples. My husband, Larry, assists me as we help husbands and wives work through past mistakes or abuse. Marriages improve as spouses work on their own lives.

The ladies and men come to the post-abortion classes with trepidation. They don't know what to expect. I start every group knowing God will work in each life that opens up to Him. By the end of the fourteen-week study, class members understand themselves better, understand God's character better, have made new friends, and have found their investment of time was well worth it.

I led the **Free Me to Live** Bible study by Ken Freeman for six years, and I felt it was an awesome privilege. I met marvelous people who trusted me with the skeletons in their closets. They allowed me to enter into their deepest hurts. I witnessed God's love and forgiveness transforming lives. I, too, let go of hurts from my own past and forgave abusers. I discovered new depths of God's love and forgiveness, and I'm grateful I had this opportunity to participate in God's healing the lives of hurting people.

Second Chances

by Jami Sims

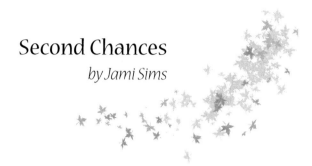

Early one January, my ten-year-old daughter, Madelyn, and I posted flyers on the campus of Auburn University advertising a ten-week post-abortion recovery support class that I planned to lead at the Women's Hope Medical Clinic in Auburn/Opelika, Alabama. With each flyer we hung, I told Madelyn how God would use our class to lead others to Him.

Time passed, but I received no calls from the flyers. Nothing.

I knew many women needed the class because I knew how I had struggled. Lured into premarital sex by the promise of love, at seventeen I stared at two blue lines indicating a positive pregnancy test. I was petrified. Panic superseded rationale. I remember making the call to the abortion clinic as if it were yesterday. With my stomach in knots, I scheduled the appointment.

I have always believed abortion is wrong, but when I faced an unplanned and unwanted pregnancy, thoughts

Among women 25 to 44 years of age who reported having had an unintended birth (either mistimed or unwanted at time of conception) ~

About . . .
61% had less than a high school degree

18% had college degrees. [16]

79

flooded in: *This will be an easy way out. I won't have to deal with this problem. No one will ever know.*

I entered the front door of the abortion clinic and was quickly ushered out the back door, sent on my way not fully understanding what had happened to my body, heart, and soul during those brief moments I lay on the sterile table of an abortionist.

Afterwards, guilt and shame engulfed me. I coped with the emotions I was experiencing—or trying *not* to experience—by numbing myself to the world with alcohol or anything else I could get my hands on.

I didn't know this behavior could be attributed to the choice I had made. Maybe not 100 percent, but I recognized a marked difference in my behavior after my abortion. I was different.

Almost two years later I was pregnant again. Though horrified once again, I would not go through another abortion. Could this be my second chance? I would carry this baby, and it would be my redemption.

Madelyn was born December 18, 1993.

I chose abortion at seventeen and gave birth at nineteen.

I've known both sides. I have learned that death begets death and life begets life. I chose life for Madelyn, and God used her to divert me from the self-destructive path I had wandered down since the abortion. When I engaged in self-destructive behaviors, I head God whisper to my soul, *Is this the environment* you want her in? It wasn't. I now had her well-being to consider.

In 1998 I married. Reluctantly, I told my husband, Brad, of my past. He was deeply hurt, but he still loved me. I had grown up in a Christian home so I knew about forgiveness, but I didn't *feel* forgiven. Brad supported me and loved me unconditionally as I worked through denial, anger, bitterness, and finally accepting the choice I had made. The process brought wholeness

About 61% of abortions are obtained by women who have one or more children. [17]

 80

to my broken heart, and I was finally able to feel forgiven by God.

After that, I felt a tug on my heart to get involved with a local pregnancy care center. I wanted to help other women who'd been through abortion find the forgiveness, peace, and freedom I had finally found. That's what this class was designed for. Women need a safe place to get honest with themselves and with God, a place to discover that God is not mean, vindictive, or waiting to zap us—a place where they can receive forgiveness. That's so important because women who have chosen abortion often feel they have committed the unforgivable.

I wanted them to meet Jesus Christ—God in flesh. Having a relationship with Him gives me hope, victory, and purpose for this life—in the here and now. This is an inner hope, joy, and victory that no one can take away.

There had to be women on the campus of Auburn University who needed my class. We weren't seeing any response, yet I believed God would provide the women. Finally two signed up.

Then one evening another young woman called to inquire about the class. "I've seen the flyers around campus," she said, hesitantly. "Each time I saw one I became more convinced that the time has come for me to deal with my past."

She proved to be an exemplary participant. She was not a believer in the Lord Jesus Christ, but she was interested in the teachings of the Bible and the principles taught in the class. She invited me to visit her, and I found her apartment covered with Scripture verses from the class written on cards. I sensed in her an eagerness to experience freedom from her past, but I also sensed in her a reluctance to let go of the wrong thinking, self-condemnation, and self-destructive behaviors that hindered her from breaking free.

The time came for our final class. By the time we'd worked through the study, we had a lot to celebrate. There was a sense of breaking free to newfound healing and a new life. No longer did these women fear the past. And no longer did they fear the future. There was a lot to celebrate, and I had the evening all planned. Music played. We ate snacks. We laughed and joked. But not everything was going as planned.

My friend seemed sad, downcast, markedly different from the other women.

Gently, I asked her if, during the course of our class, she trusted that Jesus had paid for her sins? Had she trusted that she was truly forgiven?

Her eyes grew wet with tears. She shook her head no.

"Would you like to trust Him with that tonight?"

She closed her eyes and nodded—*Yes!*

I helped her pray a prayer expressing that very thing. As all of us sat around a table, we prayed together, admitting that we are sinners and we can't save ourselves. Together we acknowledged that Christ paid for all our sins. We confessed that we were allowing Him to be our Lord and Savior, were putting our trust and faith in Him, and wanted to build a relationship with Him. When we said "amen," everyone was excited, including my young friend! We lingered in this moment of transformation. We sensed the movement from darkness to light, from death to life.

I didn't teach that class again. It's as if God meant that class for those three ladies. Now I teach part of the training program for counselors who work at pregnancy centers, and I speak to women's groups, at fund-raisers, and in churches. And that's enough, because Brad and I now have Madelyn and seven more precious children!

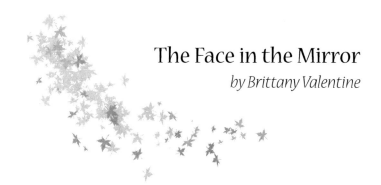

The Face in the Mirror

by Brittany Valentine

I remember the exercise as if it were yesterday. During the concluding classes for the Abortion Recovery Assistance class I had enrolled in, I was to look into the mirror at my own face. *A simple enough exercise*, I thought. *This can't possibly be all that life changing.*

My teacher rambled off instructions. When I heard my name, I went through the motions, standing up and walking to the mirror. I saw myself. Nothing different.

But as the teacher began to share that God, the Creator of the entire universe, loved me and forgave me for aborting the baby that He had given me, I lost all awareness of others in the room. The depth of God's immense love and unparalleled forgiveness had an indescribable impact on me.

Words can never describe the eternal work the Lord did in me during those few short minutes. My heart was completely overcome with the forgiveness of the cross of Jesus. The unconditional, undeserved mercy of Jesus Christ swept away my guilt and shame and I began living under "a crown of beauty instead of ashes, the oil of gladness instead of mourning," as Isaiah wrote in the Old Testament (v. 61:3).

I knew from that moment on when I heard the word *abortion*, I would no longer cringe in shame and despair. I knew my heart would glorify the Risen Savior who shed His blood to take away my shame by His amazing grace.

I still remember the moment I realized that God, knowing everything and being completely Sovereign, knew when He gave me that baby I would choose to abort the child. God knew, and yet He still gave me that child.

He taught me of His love and forgiveness in the most amazing way. So personal. So painful. Yet all the while so lovingly and gently. Being completely lost in His incomparable goodness and grace, I have no choice but to share His love.

I praise God for the work He is doing in the local women's center, the work that took me to the cross and healed my heart.

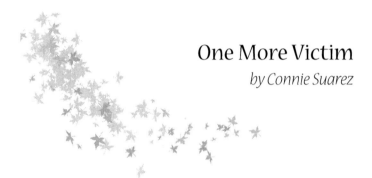

One More Victim

by Connie Suarez

When Char came to volunteer at the Arkansas Valley Pregnancy Center in La Junta, Colorado, she was not going to talk to me. She had lived her life in that mode for nearly two decades: avoiding people and situations that risked exposing her terrible secret. She certainly wasn't going to tell me or anyone else she'd had an abortion almost twenty years earlier. Char just wanted to help the pregnancy center help other women who were in the same spot she had found herself in years ago.

Char felt safe coming in that day because I wasn't supposed to be at the center. Somehow she felt her secret would be safe with the other staff, but not with the director.

But I was there that day, and Char did share with me about her past abortion.

I explained our policy required her to complete a post-abortion Bible study before she could counsel clients. I thought it would be a mere formality. Char agreed to go through the study with me.

Early in the Bible study, Char spoke with bitterness about the abortion doctor. "They had ultrasound equipment in that clinic, but they didn't use it," she said. Several years after her abortion, she was pregnant again and had an ultrasound. "I got to see the heartbeat, the little arms and legs of this baby that I wanted," she said. But there was no ultrasound with her first pregnancy. She said, "I'm sure they were afraid if I saw an ultrasound, I'd change my mind."

As we worked through the Bible study, Char bitterly recalled the events she experienced. "The day of the abortion, the doctor was very cruel," she said. "Right in front of me he told the nurse, 'We should have gotten paid twice because it was twins.' "

Char wondered how he could have known she was carrying twins since no ultrasound had been done. I knew enough about abortion procedures to guess the doctor had seen the remains of the babies that had been removed from Char's womb. Char wept bitterly whenever she talked about the incident, so I felt reluctant to add to her grief by sharing the details of an abortion.

As I met with Char, some weeks she would tense and rock back and forth as she made the hard decision to forgive someone involved with her abortion. Other weeks she struggled with the need to ask someone to forgive her for her actions. Then the day came when again she relived that awful moment when the doctor told her she had aborted two babies, not one. "Char," I began to explain as gently as I could, "someone, perhaps that doctor, had to check to make sure the entire baby had been removed. Otherwise, the mother is at risk for infection."

Tears filled Char's eyes. "He's just one more victim," she whispered. "He's not the arch-villain in my story. I didn't know what he had to do for me. He's just one more victim of abortion." Those tears filling Char's eyes were tears of compassion and forgiveness. Her stiff body softened as she realized the job that doctor performed to help her cover up her sin.

That day Char began praying for that doctor. "Lord, I pray he would no longer want to perform abortions," she prayed. "Bring him to eternal salvation in Your Son Jesus Christ."

Char still tears up when she speaks about what the doctor told her that day. She will always grieve the loss of her two precious babies. But she isn't angry or bitter with the doctor anymore. "I want the best for him," she says. "I pray for him often. It must have been an awfully difficult thing for him to have to perform abortions every day. Someday I want to meet him, whether here or in heaven. He will always have a special place in my heart."

Resources

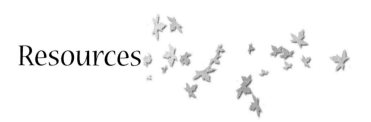

Struggling after an abortion? Find help here:

 Organizations:
- Ramah International: http://www.ramahinternational.org/ 1776 Hudson Street, Englewood, FL 34223 (941) 473-2188 Contact Sydna Masse at Sydna@aol.com.
- Rachel's Vineyard, an international post-abortion healing outreach of Priests for Life: http://www.rachelsvineyard.org/
- Silent No More Awareness: http://www.silentnomoreawareness.org/search/
- Operation Outcry: http://www.operationoutcry.org/pages.asp?pageid=23064

 Especially for men:
- Rachel's Vineyard, an international post-abortion healing outreach of Priests for Life, web page for men: http://www.rachelsvineyard.org/men/
- http://www.fatherhoodforever.org/

 Help by e-mail:
- Free e-mail course, *Free Me to Live*, at http://www.freemetolive.com/.

Information on Post-Abortion Syndrome and symptoms:
- http://www.sbpcc.net/post-abortion_help.htm
- http://postabortionsyndrome.org/post_abortion_syndrome _symptoms.html

 Information on Abortion's link to breast cancer:
- Breast Cancer Prevention Institute: http://bcpinstitute.org/home.htm
- Printable pamphlet in PDF: http://bcpinstitute.org/BreastCancerRisksPrevention_4ed.pdf

 Books:
- ***Forgiven and Set Free:*** *A Post-Abortion Bible Study for Women* by Linda Cochrane (Baker, 1999)
- ***Redeeming a Father's Heart:*** *Men Share Powerful Stories of Abortion Loss and Recovery* (AuthorHouse, 2007).
- ***Her Choice to Heal:*** *Finding Spiritual and Emotional Peace After Abortion* by Sydna Masse and Joan Phillips (Chariot Victor/Cook, 1998)
- ***Won by Love:*** *Norma McCorvey, Jane Roe of Roe v. Wade, Speaks Out for the Unborn As She Shares Her New Conviction for Life* by Norma McCorvey and Gary Thomas (Nelson, 1998)

DVDs:

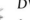

- **Faces of Abortion**, originally for TV is now available on DVD. Joyce Zounis ("Multiple Mercies") has hosted and produced this television show and Tina Brock ("It's Never Over") has been a guest on the show. Their stories appear above.

- **I Was Wrong** features Norma McCorvey, "Jane Roe" of the Supreme Court case Roe v. Wade, and Joyce Zounis, whose story "Multiple Mercies" appears in this chapter.

Music:

- **The Choice** by Chris Jackman (see her story "The Choice" in this chapter) is available only through Abortion Recovery InterNational. http://www.abortionrecoveryinternational.org/ (Click "Resources.")

- "A Baby's Prayer" by Kathy Troccoli is on her **Love and Mercy** CD (Reunion, 1997).

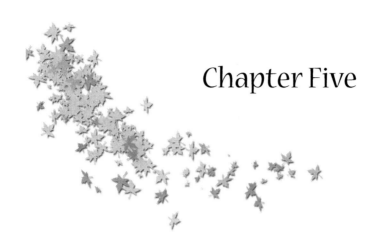

Chapter Five

For, By, and About Men

I love the LORD, for he heard my voice,
he heard my cry for mercy. PSALM 116:1

Is unplanned pregnancy just a "woman's issue"?

For every pregnancy, there is a daddy. What about the men?

Men often feel—or are made to feel—that they have no say in what choice a woman makes for her pregnancy. He may tell her it's up to her; whatever she wants to do. Or he may push for one choice or another.

In his, "Whatever you want to do," he may intend to be supportive. He may want to see his child brought into the world. He may want to raise his child. He may secretly be terrified and fear becoming a daddy. He may be a lot of things.

And how does he sound to her? If he says the decision is all up to her, is she wondering if he'll support her if she keeps the child? And if a man indicates he doesn't want her to keep the child, would she find it hard to fight against him knowing she then may have to go it alone—without him?

Many people may think unplanned pregnancy is a woman's issue. But here are stories from, by, and about the men. These men share their stories of unplanned pregnancy, the choices they made, and how it all affected them. Hear what these men have to say, now that they've had time to contemplate their choices and to live with the decisions that they made.

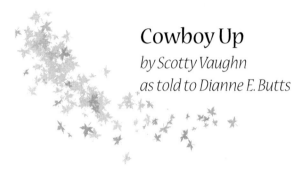

Cowboy Up

by Scotty Vaughn
as told to Dianne E. Butts

I was a road musician, married, and we already had two children when we learned my wife was pregnant again. In the circle of folks I hung with, we made agreements with the world, and the world said abortion was just a choice. It was another form of birth control. We even had a pastor at the church we went to agree with us saying, "This is not a good time for you to have another child."

My wife, to her credit, didn't want an abortion. My parents said, "This is not something you want to do."

But I was young and arrogant, and it was my way or the highway. I didn't really consider my wife's perspective at all. I was the driving force behind the abortion.

In my twenties I did it all. You know: drugs, alcohol . . . My first wife and I eventually divorced. I slept around . . .

After I turned thirty I started trying to straighten my life up. Most of what I did, the glaring wrong choices I was making, came to a head when I became a Christian. But not this one. It was still several years after I became a Christian before I was

Of all abortions, married women obtain 18.4%. [1]

92

sitting in a church service where the pastor preached a sermon on Psalm 139, which in part says:

> For you created my inmost being; you knit me together in my mother's womb. I praise you because I am fearfully and wonderfully made; your works are wonderful, I know that full well.
>
> My frame was not hidden from you when I was made in the secret place. When I was woven together in the depths of the earth, your eyes saw my unformed body.
>
> All the days ordained for me were written in your book before one of them came to be. (Psalm 139:13–16)

That sermon, and the words of the psalmist talking to God, opened up more than I could even begin to handle. I went into denial and didn't deal with any of it.

One night, I woke up to a "voice"—probably not an audible voice because I had remarried and my wife, Cindy, was lying right there beside me and she didn't hear it. But it was audible to me.

I kept hearing, "Your spiritual act of worship. . . . This is your spiritual act of worship" echoing over and over.

After I came to Christ, one Bible verse especially pulled me out of the pit. It's Romans 12:1: "Therefore, I urge you, brothers, in view of God's mercy, to offer your bodies as living sacrifices, holy and pleasing to God—this is your spiritual act of worship." This had been my prayer, my commitment to God. And now that last phrase was echoing back to me.

I knew God was in the room with me that night. He was letting me know there was a lot more going on than I knew. He was speaking to me, but I didn't understand what He was saying right away.

Shortly after that my first grandchild was born. I picked Shelby up in my arms and held that beautiful little baby girl, and I felt overwhelming joy. Then all the sudden I was absolutely devastated. Because I knew. I knew.

I couldn't hide after that. I couldn't go away and not deal with it. Thank God, by then He had given me some spiritual understanding, so I knew I had to get on my knees and do some business with God.

It took quite a while. For a couple weeks I just cried over the whole thing. I pictured my baby—that baby we had aborted—in Jesus' arms. I was absolutely devastated. Fathers are supposed to die for their children, not the other way around.

I had a strong sense that my child had been a little baby girl. I named her Janey.

Through the birth of my next two grandchildren I felt almost like I was Peter at the lake. After Peter had denied Jesus three times, the resurrected Jesus asked Peter three times, "Do you love Me?" When Peter answered yes, Jesus said, "Then feed my sheep." My first three grandchildren were all little girls—Shelby, then Halle and Gracie—and I felt Him saying, "If you love Me, then love these little babies."

Then one morning, TV news was covering a women's march for "Choice." It brought back that sick-to-my-stomach-because-of-the-abortion feeling. I got in my truck, drove across town, found Life Network in Colorado Springs, walked in, and told those folks, "I gotta talk to somebody." Those folks helped me work through what I had done.

I learned some things going through that. I learned that first, you gotta come out of denial. You gotta own it. If you don't own it, it will own you.

And once you come to grips with what you've done, you're going to get pounded with shame and guilt. Those are all stages of grief. But we, as men, don't think we're supposed to be able to feel this grief.

I don't think there really is healing for this in this world apart from healing from God. In the New Testament we read that Saul probably held the coats of those who stoned Stephen to death, the first Christian to die for Christ. Saul probably stood close enough that Stephen's blood splattered on him. Didn't I stand there and hold that doctor's coat while he took the life of my

 94

child? That's not a fun place to go. But it was there that God found Saul and not only gave him forgiveness and grace—that unconditional, undeserved total love from God—but calling. Saul became Paul, the Apostle.

I've learned our point of greatest failing is often where God calls us to do His work. For years I worked as an emcee and storyteller at the famous Flying W Ranch in Colorado Springs, Colorado. Now I'm the pastor of the ranch's Cowboy Church. And I have my ministry called "Cowboy Up" where I work with post-abortive men. I speak all around the country sharing my story. To "cowboy up" is not doing what the world says we should do: "Just forget about it." Cowboy up means, "Be man enough to *not* forget about it."

Most of the stories I've read say the man didn't have a choice; the woman made the decision and moved on. Certainly there are stories like that, but to be honest, in my experience working with men I haven't seen that very often. Most of the time I see one of two scenarios:

The man told the woman, "You just do whatever you want to do." In other words, he checked out. He didn't offer her his strength. When we say, "You make your own decision," we're saying, "I don't want any part of this."

A post-abortive father can fall into several groups:

- He insisted or forced his wife or girlfriend to have an abortion.

- He allowed his wife or girlfriend to make the decision to abort.

- He didn't want the abortion to take place and tried to actively stop it.

- He found out about the abortion after it was completed and had no voice in the decision. [2]

At current rates, by age 45, about 43% of all women will have at least one abortion. [3]

Or the man is just like me and either subtly, or not so subtly said, "This is a problem. This is an imposition. You need to get rid of this baby."

Unfortunately our society today tells us that men are bad if we take a stand. But we struggle because the sanctity of life is written into the fabric of who we are as men: we are protectors. Abortion is a direct attack on our identity as protector of our children.

Statistics say one out of every three women in the church has had an abortion.

That's over 50 million since *Roe versus Wade* legalized abortion on demand in 1973.[4] But every number you see is about women. Well, women didn't do this all by themselves. Men seem invisible in this issue, but I know one out of every three *men* in the church are post-abortive as well. So much of the focus is on getting to the women to save the babies, but we need to save them all. The men and women who have experienced abortion need saved, too.

Janey is a part of my family now. I was able to talk with my parents about her before they died. I was able to say to my Dad while he was in a coma, "Dad, when you get there, your little baby granddaughter is going to be there." I don't know that she'll be a baby, but I knew my Dad would know her. Janey, and the fact that she's now with God, is very real to me. She's a part of my life.

I learned that I could start making Janey's life count. I began working with Life Network, in Colorado Springs. I teach post-abortive Bible studies, like *Healing the Father's Heart*. And I work with Life Steps to mentor young couples who are making those decisions. Most of the time they're not married but are living together and don't have any kind of religious faith—and that's fine. They don't need to be Christians to come in to see us. No matter who they are, I'll work with them and walk beside them and mentor them and help them.

I've also learned God doesn't call us *to* brokenness, but *through* brokenness. Brokenness is a place on the trip, but at the cross of Christ there is restoration. If you'll understand and embrace your loss, then Jesus will go through that with you. Then He will empower you to help other people make different choices.

Scotty Vaughn isn't alone in his struggles after abortion. Dan Ambrecht also works to help others heal after the choices they've made.

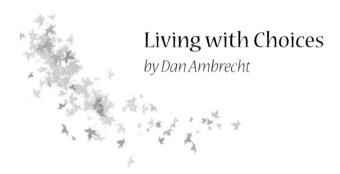

Living with Choices
by Dan Ambrecht

Standing outside the busy pregnancy medical clinic where I was executive director, I visited with the chairman of our board. We talked about the nature of pro-life work, issues of managing the pregnancy center, theology . . . whatever came up. It was hot as we stood under a palm tree across the small street from our front door. Cars passed on the street and pulled up in front of the building at the end of the street. Doors opened and women were helped gently into the cars. We watched the comings and goings at the abortion provider that shared our street.

I was in full-time pro-life work, but abortionists everywhere were still busy. Women and their families were making decisions of life and death with too little information. My heart ached for them.

But I was surprised to realize I had little feeling for the babies that had been lost in that place. That concerned me. My very purpose when entering pro-life work was to save the babies. They were innocent; God had a plan for their lives.

God knew what the outcome would be when they were conceived. Still, I don't believe His intent was ever for them to be aborted.

Why was I not thinking of those babies? I wondered. I wrestled with that for some time. *Lord, what would you have me do?* I prayed. I didn't know what else to do. *Lord, please be with those women visiting the abortionists. Watch over them and their families. Draw them closer to You through the ordeal they've chosen.*

But what about the babies?

My heart ached for the women and for the men who believed, as I did long ago, that an abortion would solve their problem. But why was I not troubled about the babies?

Then it came to me: they were safe in Jesus' arms. For the mothers, the difficulty, the challenges, the questioning of their decision was only beginning. For the fathers, trying to hide from their role in it was only beginning.

For me, it was an awakening. Despite my desire to save babies from the fate of abortion, that was only part of my mission. The rest of it was to care for those who made the decision that I had made so many years before.

My partnership with God grew with that realization. My job was to pray, listen carefully, and to be on task. His job was to save the babies that could be saved. My job was to, with prayer, minister to those living with their choices.

Josh* and Amy* struggled as a couple after their unplanned pregnancy. They allowed Carol McGalliard to tell us their story.

Life After Abortion

by Carol McGalliard

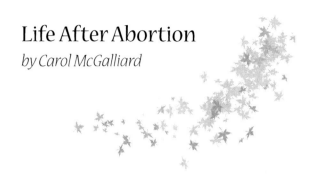

Josh* was a seminary student when his girlfriend, Amy,* learned she was pregnant. Neither of them had jobs, and they believed they could not support a child. Also, because they were not married, they knew Josh's future in Christian ministry would be jeopardized, so they decided to abort. One week later, Josh drove Amy to an abortion clinic that helped them carry out their decision.

Some men and women report an initial relief following an abortion. Josh and Amy did not. "I knew we had made a mistake the minute Amy walked out of the recovery room," Josh said. "The look on her face— Already I wanted to go back. What I had done hit me hard. I will always be the guy who killed his own kid.

"After that, I became very secretive."

Amy was nearly hysterical when they left the clinic. "The sadness after the abortion was crushing," she says. "That was the day I started feeling defeated and angry."

Talking about the abortion was so painful that Josh and Amy gave up after a few attempts. Both kept all the hurt, anger, and despair bottled up inside. Neither of them anticipated how devastating the secret and unresolved emotions would be to their relationship. Their relationship became very volatile. Still, they later married.

The birth of their son did nothing to heal their emotions or their marriage.

"When our son was born," Josh said, "I freaked. I would picture myself throwing him out the window or over the rail. I couldn't figure out why I had these thoughts because I certainly had no intention of doing these things. In other situations, I would panic and become too protective. I never told anyone about this for fear they would think I was crazy."

Amy uses one word to describe their marriage: miserable. She criticized Josh and they fought constantly. She was plagued with mouth ulcers. She doubted her ability to be a good wife and mother. She second-guessed her decisions. To relieve her stress and anger, Amy began drinking. She had no confidence in herself to make the marriage work, so she left Josh and filed for divorce.

After the separation, Amy formed a deep bond of friendship with her mother. As Amy's trust in her mother grew, she found the courage to tell her mother her deepest secret. "When my mother did not condemn me," Amy said, "I experienced the relief the psalmist describes: 'When I kept silent my bones wasted away. . . . Then I acknowledged my sin to you . . . and you forgave the guilt of my sin' (Psalm 32:3, 5).

Amy's mother encouraged her to get involved in a post-abortion group. "I joined PACE (Post Abortion Counseling and Education)," she said. "At PACE I began my journey through the healing process. The steps to healing were: telling your story (confession), mourning the loss, grieving the sin, and receiving God's forgiveness. I was apprehensive about telling the group that I had participated in killing my child. I feared condemnation and rejection, but the PACE staff offered me grace. They did not minimize what I had done, but the PACE leaders taught about grace for the repentant. They taught about God's holiness and about His love and His acceptance of us in spite of our sin.

"When I attended PACE," Amy continued, "for the first time, I found hope that I could live without being angry and bitter, hope that I could resolve my marriage problems. I allowed myself to be sad for what I'd lost—my child. I realized I had lived in a prison of anger and bitterness, and that the anger had been a cover-up for guilt and sadness. I was angry because Josh had not been strong; he had not protected me or our child. Because I had not acknowledged my sin, my anger found other reasons to surface, and Josh was usually the victim of that anger.

"As I studied the Bible, I realized the magnitude of what abortion is in the eyes of a Holy God. The counselor taught me from Scripture that I am forgiven. But it was the grace she and my mom extended to me that softened my heart. Receiving God's forgiveness gave me strength to forgive Josh. I mourned deeply for the loss of my child. It was terribly painful. But as I worked through the grief, my anger began to dissipate. Both the sin and the loss were exposed, so I no longer needed anger to cover up the guilt and hurt. I was no longer held captive by a secret."

During the separation, Josh attended counseling and began dealing with his post-abortion issues. When each of them began to heal from the ordeal, they found reconciliation not divorce was a natural part of the healing process. Josh and Amy prayed together. They mourned together. "When we acknowledged we had killed our child, we were able to resolve the pent-up feelings that had caused our problems," Amy said. "We were able to begin rebuilding our marriage."

After Josh and Amy reconciled, Josh began volunteering at the local pregnancy care clinic, Hope Pregnancy Center of Brazos Valley, Texas. Volunteers are required to go through a training program.

"In this program," Josh said, "I learned that my problems stemmed from the abortion of my child. It's hard to admit that one day you were not a man. Instead, you were a coward and did not protect your child. There was help available through the church or my parents. If I could have seen pictures showing the baby's development in the womb when it is only a few weeks old, I don't think we would have done it. I take full responsibility for the decision. It's a horrible story, a perspective I wish I didn't have, but Romans 8:28 says God can use all things to bring something good.

"I have spoken publically of my abortion experience. Each time I talk about it, I relive forgiveness and grace all over again. It's good to think about what abortion is. You linked yourself to murder, but when you face the pain of that, God's grace is pretty unreal."

Mouth ulcers no longer plague Amy, and she no longer drinks to suppress painful emotions. Josh takes the initiative for the family to read Scripture together, to pray, and worship together. Amy sees tenderness in Josh as he protects her and their children.

Their pastor, their parents, and their friends all say they see a major change in both Josh and Amy, and in their relationship. The constant conflict, the anger and bitterness are gone. Josh and Amy say they know they are forgiven. "We are freed from the prison of secrecy and anger—freed to become the joy-filled man and woman God created us to be." Josh and Amy found there is life after abortion.

Ed* is a man who was deeply affected by unplanned pregnancy . . . in more ways than one. Here is his story:

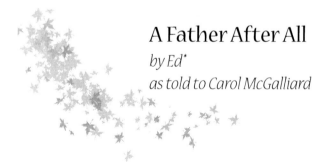

A Father After All
by Ed*
as told to Carol McGalliard

"Make love, not war" echoed on the campus and city streets when I arrived at college in the early 1970s. Tie-dyed shirts, faded jeans, and peace signs dotted the campus, and "free love" was the call of the day. Soon I was living with a girl I met there at college. When we learned she was pregnant, we knew we were not serious enough about our relationship to consider marriage. Abortion wasn't yet legal, but there were "semi-legal" ways around this obstacle. If you consulted the right psychiatrist, who knew the right physician, you could get an abortion for "psychological" reasons.

While my girlfriend underwent the procedure, I sat in a bar a few blocks away drinking alone, trying to drown the reality of the wrong being done to my child. *I will probably never have kids,* I thought. *I will never be a father.*

Like many couples involved in an abortion, my girlfriend and I soon parted. My involvement in drugs and "free love" deepened with time. I lived with an older woman who had two teenagers. Our involvement in the drinking and drug culture intensified until we had no friends who weren't addicts. I began longing for a different life.

While clerking at a convenience store in my neighborhood, I met a man who was instrumental in helping me begin to find the different life I longed for. He was a customer who just walked into the store one day and began asking me what I believed about God and heaven. The man returned several times to talk with me. Soon I was visiting him and his wife in their home. We read and discussed the Bible and prayed together. Shortly after, I asked Christ to be my Savior.

I did as the man recommended and began reading the Bible. I devoured it, amazed by the healing I found there. I had been drinking lots of alcohol daily, but I simply quit. My desire for it was gone. I found real peace in knowing I was forgiven for everything—the drugs, the drinking, the sex outside of marriage . . . and the abortion.

The woman I lived with liked the changes she saw in me and, without any pressure from me, began to ask questions about my faith. Within a few weeks, she too became a Christian and we were married.

I went back to that neighbor's home to share the good news with him and his wife, but the man had vanished from the neighborhood. None of the neighbors could recall seeing anyone living at the house where I had visited and prayed with this Christian man.

Sometime later, my stepdaughter, Karen,* became pregnant. Because she was using drugs, her doctor recommended abortion. He believed the baby would be severely damaged by her drug use. In fact, he and his staff went beyond recommending abortion—they pressured Karen, implying she would be doing the baby a favor because it could never have a normal life. When she asked about consulting another doctor, they told her she would never find a doctor who would take her as a patient because of her drug use. Abortion was no big deal according to them. Since she had already been through one abortion, Karen knew it was a big deal and wanted no part of a second.

I prayed with her and encouraged her to stand her ground. I found a doctor in another state who specialized in helping addicts through pregnancy and delivery. With this doctor's help, Karen carried her baby to full term and delivered a healthy baby boy, Sam.*

There were no developmental problems of any kind with the baby. He has grown into a bright young man who enrolled in college and is working toward his career goals. And he walks with the Lord.

Karen continued to struggle with drugs, so me and my wife raised Sam. We are not related genetically, but Sam is my son. He calls me Dad. I could not love him more. Raising him was not a chore—it was a privilege. In Sam, God gave back the precious life I destroyed with abortion.

I guess I've played two major roles in Sam's life: first, as his advocate while he was still in the womb. Then as his father, providing for him and protecting him, but most importantly pointing him to the heavenly Father. In spite of my mistakes, I am a father after all.

My own involvement in abortion was not the main catalyst that led me to volunteer with the local pregnancy care center. My main motivation was Karen's struggle. Even though Karen did not want an abortion, the pressure she felt was almost more than she could endure. As I watched physicians and nurses pressure her to abort, I ached for the young woman I loved as my daughter. The people who had studied and trained to preserve life and bring healing pressured her to end the life of her child. I believed this was wrong. My anger led me to become involved in helping men and women faced with the crisis created by an unwanted pregnancy. I encourage them to preserve the life of their unborn child, and I help them prepare to care for the child.

In addition to counseling with men at the center, I also tend the grounds and do repairs, anything I can do to help cut costs. My aim is to create a pleasant environment for people who come needing help with an unplanned pregnancy.

I know I'm forgiven. Helping at the center is not about working to make up for the wrong I did. Jesus Christ did that. I am trying to show the love of God by giving others the help and guidance I didn't have when I faced that same situation.

How many times have we heard "it's not a baby, it's a cluster of cells" or something similar? Jim Schultz believed that for fifteen years. And then it took another seven for him to find relief from the guilt and shame he experienced. Here is Jim's story.

Life is Precious
by Jim Schultz
as told to Helen Hoover

While moseying past various booths set up by the local merchants and civic organizations at our town's Fall Festival, my wife and I came to a crisis pregnancy center's booth. We stopped to chat with the lady. She explained their purpose was to educate the public, and any woman who came to the center for a free pregnancy test, concerning abortion, adoption, and parenting. She then showed us pictures of the stages and growth of a fetus from conception until birth.

My thoughts were a jumble. I flashed back fifteen years. *It wasn't a blob, but a life! How could I have agreed for my girlfriend to have an abortion? Why hadn't I realized it was a baby growing in her? Oh no, I allowed my baby to be killed for convenience!* Guilt, shame, and sorrow immediately surfaced.

After we arrived back home, my wife and I talked about what we had learned about abortion and the development of a fetus. My wife had an abortion when she was a teenager. Now we both realized we had issues connected with the abortions in our lives, but we didn't know what to do about them.

Time passed. Then one day, seven years after we'd talked with that lady at the Fall Festival, my wife said, "I heard that crisis pregnancy center is offering a Bible study for couples to deal with abortion issues. We've been looking for answers to our problems associated with the abortions. How about we attend?"

I readily agreed . . . um, so I could help my wife with her issues. I never expected to be touched by God myself. The study was called *Free Me to Live* by Ken Freeman. We met weekly for twelve weeks. Besides the discussion and exercises during class time, we each had homework. As we explored the Bible, our sometimes incorrect beliefs about God and His character were challenged. The study dealt with issues about the abortion and abuse, and we studied God's love, grace, mercy, reconciliation, and forgiveness.

We read and studied many Scriptures to bring us to the realization of God's forgiveness. We were encouraged to accept His forgiveness for us, forgive others for what they had done to us, and forgive ourselves. Seeing God's full forgiveness, even for an abortion, allowed me to start thinking how each and every life is precious.

One evening the leader handed out small white rocks with a permanent marker. She prayed that God would reveal to each participant any situation or person that was weighing us down.

As God revealed situations to us, we wrote each one on a rock. We put the rocks in a small rough burlap bag and were told to hang the bag over our shoulder to represent the burden that those things were to us. Then we went to a river.

The leader told us, "Look at each rock individually and forgive the person or situation. Then throw it as far as you can into the river." That was a freeing exercise.

Another evening we made a collage. The group leader gave us a piece of construction paper and a magazine. She told us, "As you thumb through the magazine, cut out any pictures or words that stand out to you. Paste any number of pictures on your construction paper and then we'll look at them."

Some of the other participants had several pictures of children, scenery, houses, and words. Each person deciphered their collage, with insights from the leader and the rest of us.

On my paper I had three pictures. My wife and I each have three children from previous marriages so I immediately knew that the two pictures of three children each represented our children. But then, down in the corner, was a picture of a little girl. I was puzzled, until someone suggested that maybe this was the aborted child.

"Yes, that's it," I said.

The collage represented all the children in my life. The picture of the little girl brought recognition to the baby I'd agreed to have aborted. Before the Bible study was finished, I named the little girl Micayla.

I had many more issues about the abortion than I had realized when I started the Bible study. I now could feel God's forgiveness instead of the guilt or shame that the devil put on me.

The last night of the Bible study we had a memorial service in a local church. This gave me the opportunity to remember Micayla in a forgiven way instead of with guilt attached.

That collage is now framed and hangs in our home. It is a reminder of God's forgiveness and of the precious life, who now resides in heaven.

Before taking that Bible study, I didn't see how precious children are. I couldn't because of the guilt, shame, and sorrow in my life. I am glad to have overcome the bad issues associated with the death of my precious little girl. I now know that God sees each life as precious, and so do I. And I continue to live under God's grace and mercy through His freedom. I am indeed free to live.

Having an abortion in the past is not the only reason men come into pregnancy centers. Oddie had other reasons for entering a pregnancy center, among them simply wanting to be a good father.

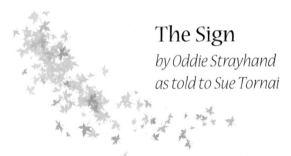

The Sign
by Oddie Strayhand as told to Sue Tornai

My girlfriend, April, didn't know for sure if she was pregnant. We were afraid and didn't know who we could talk to. April finally talked with one of her friends at work.

"I drive by this place every day," her friend said. "A sign outside says 'Free Pregnancy Test.'"

"Are you sure?" April asked. "Do you remember the name of the place?"

"No," she said, "but it's at El Camino and Fulton. You can't miss it."

April and I took a day off work and we went to check out this place. The name on the door was "Alternatives Pregnancy Resource Center." As soon as we entered we felt loved by everyone there. At first we were uncomfortable and nervous about sharing our situation with a bunch of strangers, but we connected with Flavia right away. We were able to talk openly with her without feeling judged.

I was excited when Flavia told us April's test results were positive. But I didn't know anything about pregnant women or babies. It was like Flavia read my mind. She introduced us to an education and parenting program, "Earn While You Learn."

April and I didn't expect anything from the Center. We thought we would get a pregnancy test and that would be it. We didn't know we could get hands-on training and earn "Mommy Bucks" to shop in the Nursery Nook. It's the best program! Our assignments helped me learn how to help April and how to be a good father. There was a lot of stuff I didn't know. The lessons kept my interest, and they were intriguing and informative. I thoroughly enjoyed each class.

I remember one of our homework assignments was to write a letter to our baby. At the time we didn't know if we were having a boy or girl. We picked the name Isaiah for a boy and Nevaeh (which is "heaven" spelled backwards) for a girl. I tried to write to both, but I'll be honest with you, this letter was to Isaiah. I told him how I was looking forward to holding him. I wanted him to know he was a dream come true for me. As long as I am around, I will make sure that nothing will ever hurt him.

ODDIE'S LETTER:

Dear Isaiah or Nevaeh,
We are waiting in anticipation for you to come out and bless us as our first child. Words cannot describe the love I have for you. You are a gift from God and I plan to love and cherish you to the best of my ability.

You haven't even been born yet, but a tremendous amount of people already love and adore you. I love you and intend to teach you all I know and try my best to keep you from harm or pain.

Once again, I love you and I can't wait to finally see you!
Love,
Daddy

I love everything about being a father. Today April and I are married, and we have two sons, Isaiah and Malachi. I love spending quality time with them, even when they cry. I can't expect to be with them only when they're happy and when they want to play with me. I want to be there to calm them when they are cranky.

It's a special time for me when I get home and I see the boys smile up at me. It could be the worst day at work, but I forget everything when I see my boys.

None of this would have been possible if it wasn't for the sign that said "Free Pregnancy Test." We went for the test, and we found love and support. Now we are reaping the rewards of parenthood. It seems like our children give us much more love than we could ever give to them and we are thankful.

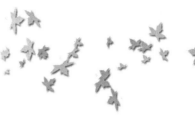

Resources

 Especially for men:
• Silent No More Awareness for men:
http://silentnomoreawareness.org/men/index.html
• Rachel's Vineyard, an international post-abortion healing outreach of Priests For Life:
http://www.rachelsvineyard.org/men/
http://www.fatherhoodforever.org/
http://www.lifeissues.org/men/Resources.html

***Information on Post-Abortion Syndrome
and symptoms:***
http://www.sbpcc.net/post-abortion_help.htm
http://postabortionsyndrome.org/post_abortion_syndrome_symptoms.html

Help for Post-Abortion Syndrome and symptoms by e-mail:

• Free e-mail course, *Free Me to Live,* at http://www.freemetolive.com/.
Healing Hearts Ministries, online study for men titled, *Wounded Warrior: Help for men suffering from Post-Abortion Trauma* www.HealingHearts.org (253) 268-0348
• *Missing Arrows,* a downloadable Bible study for men: http://www.lifeissues.org/men/missingarrows.pdf.

Books:

• *Healing a Father's Heart: A Post-Abortion Bible Study for Men* by Linda Cochrain and Kathy Jones (Baker, 1996).
• *Redeeming a Father's Heart: Men Share Powerful Stories of Abortion Loss and Recovery* (AuthorHouse, 2007).
• *David's Harp: A Daily Devotional for Post-Abortive Men by* Richard Beattie. Available from Ramah International http://ramahinternational.org/ or 1776 Hudson Street, Englewood, FL 34223 (941) 473-2188. Look for this book on the Resources page.

Addictions or troubling prenatal diagnoses:

In Ed's* story, "A Father After All," Ed told us about his daughter who struggled with addiction while she was pregnant. If someone you know is in a similar situation, has other special circumstances, or received a troubling prenatal diagnosis for the baby, you can find help from pro-life medical professionals. See the list in the Resources section at the end of chapter 8.

Other:

National Fatherhood Initiative www.fatherhood.org

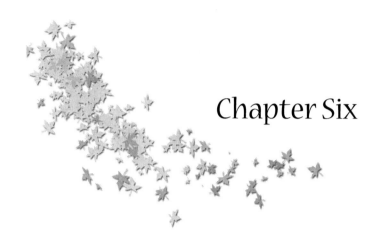

Chapter Six

Helping Her Keep Her Child

*Because he turned his ear to me,
I will call on him as long as I live..*
PSALM 116:2

When a woman wants to keep her child, those who have gone before can show her the way. Watch as the women in the following stories find the help they need. Learn where they found it and the options they discovered, even for victims of rape and incest.

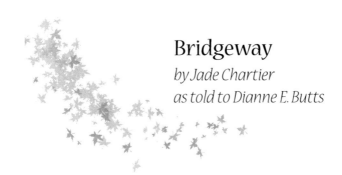

Bridgeway

by Jade Chartier
as told to Dianne E. Butts

When my biker girlfriends and I, donning our black leathers and toting baby shower gifts, walked into Bridgeway, a home for pregnant teenage girls in Lakewood, Colorado, we never expected to see a familiar face. We host a baby shower at Bridgeway two or three times each year for all the new moms and moms-to-be. It took a while, but we finally figured out who that familiar face belonged to. It was Amber.*

Several months earlier my biker girlfriends and I had visited a home for abused and neglected children. The kids instantly loved us and our black leathers and big motorcycles. One of my friends, Kristin,* formed a friendship with Amber. They shared e-mail addresses and stayed in touch. Then Amber disappeared. Kristin hadn't heard from her. We all hoped things had worked out with her family and that she had gone home. Here it was four months later and we were throwing another baby shower at Bridgeway. That's when we discovered Amber hadn't gone home. She was pregnant and now living at Bridgeway.

When Amber saw our motorcycles and black leathers, she instantly recognized us and rushed to greet us. "I lost your e-mail address," she told Kristin, "so I couldn't write and tell you where I was."

Bridgeway was founded in 1986 and allows girls to stay eighteen months from when they move in. While she lives there, Bridgeway requires each resident to attend high school or work toward her GED. When she attains a high school diploma or GED, or if she already has one, she is required to either continue

 114

her education, work at a job, or both for a minimum of twenty hours per week. Each resident has her own assigned chores, and most share a room with another mom and her baby. Every Tuesday all residents are required to attend evening activities, which include classes with life lessons, programs with speakers, or the bimonthly baby shower. Bridgeway pairs every girl with a "Bridger" or mentor.

My group of biker ladies and I are all members of the international organization Christian Motorcyclists Association. We always give each mom a Bible that has her name embossed on the cover. Inside, we highlight Bible verses especially for her.

Whenever Bridgeway throws a shower, the girls' families are always invited and often bring more gifts. At my first Bridgeway baby shower years ago, I met two young ladies: April* and Maggie.* April was about sixteen, dressed completely in black, had dyed her hair black, and was very into Goth. She was not happy her mother and older sister had come to the shower. When she unwrapped the gift her mom had brought and discovered it was a beautiful pink dress for her baby, April didn't want it. "You cannot dress your baby in black," her sister said.

"Yes I can," April said.

Meanwhile, April's friend Maggie, an eighteen-year-old, was unwrapping her gifts while her mother and aunt looked on. We bring several gifts for each girl: a gift card to a local discount department store, a disposable camera, a photo album, and a handmade baby blanket knit by a volunteer just for a particular resident at Bridgeway. Then Maggie unwrapped the Bible. "Look, Mom," she said. "It has my name on it!" Maggie had grown up in a happy, church-going Christian family. But she got pregnant and asked Bridgeway to take her in. When she thumbed through the Bible, she was amazed someone had written in it. I told her it was okay to write in the Bible. Doing so helps me remember things and find them again.

Six months later when we rode our motorcycles back to Bridgeway for another shower, April exclaimed, "You're back!" and she and Maggie ran to show us their babies. Maggie had a little boy. April had a little girl—dressed in color. April, too, was dressed in color, and she wore a beautiful smile. We couldn't believe it was the same girl. If it wasn't for her hair still dyed black, we wouldn't have recognized her. She was totally different. She said she'd been reading her Bible.

Years after I met April and Maggie, now it was Amber we were befriending and bringing gifts and a Bible to. A few months after we reconnected with her at Bridgeway, she delivered a healthy baby.

Bridgeway's motto is, "Helping pregnant teens build a new life for themselves and their children" and, to date, it has helped almost six hundred young women do just that. Bridgeway will be celebrating its twenty-fifth anniversary next year.

Would you like to visit another home that helps women in unplanned pregnancies? Welcome! Step inside the Lighthouse . . .

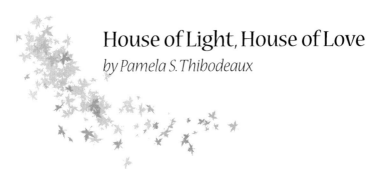

House of Light, House of Love
by Pamela S. Thibodeaux

In the rural community of Reeves, Louisiana, you would expect to see cows and horses grazing or children playing, but you wouldn't expect to see a lighthouse marking the entrance onto a forty-acre homesite nestled among pine and oak trees. But that's what you'll find.

When asked why she chose the Lighthouse for the name of her establishment, Patsy Cavenah, founder and director of Lighthouse Ministries, Inc., says, "The song 'The Lighthouse' has always ministered to me." She founded the Lighthouse in June 2001 to provide a healthy, loving, and safe environment to unwed mothers who are victims of rape, incest, abuse, and neglect. Lighthouse Ministries, Inc., is a nonprofit organization whose mission statement is the verse in the Bible Jeremiah 29:11: " 'For I know the plans I have for you,' declares the Lord, 'plans to prosper you and not to harm you, plans to give you hope and a future.' " Hope and a future are exactly what the Lighthouse provides. Since it's inception in 2001, Patsy and her staff have helped over one hundred girls.

The Lighthouse began as an old, run-down home owned by the Allen Parish School Board. The home was purchased and moved onto Patsy's property, then remodeled and restored into a dream house. The home contains two bedrooms with three twin beds in each and houses six girls at a time. Each stays free of charge throughout her pregnancy. Every girl who keeps her baby goes out on her own with resources, such as a job, or is restored to her family who then continues to shape her life. Those who place their babies for adoption are allowed to remain at The Lighthouse for an extended period to work through the grieving process and decide what to do with the remainder of their lives.

When young women enter The Lighthouse, they encounter unconditional love, hope for a better life, and God's merciful kindness. For many, it is the first time in their lives to experience any of these, much less all three. By caring for these young women and instilling in them the need for education while building their self-esteem and confidence, the staff has watched them become productive citizens in their communities.

Although adoption is a choice for the girls, no mother is forced to give up her child. Classes in childbirth, child care, breast feeding, parenting, self-esteem, etiquette, sewing, and preparation for GED along with practical life skills are offered to each girl in the home. They are also taught about the Bible.

"It is amazing to watch the transformation of those who want to change," says Patsy. "And it is our goal to see the cycle of defeat broken and the girls restored emotionally, physically, and spiritually."

Patsy recalls one twenty-one-year-old girl who had suffered abuse and so moved into drug addiction and depression. After entering the home, Patsy and the staff witnessed the complete transformation of her life. She chose adoption as the best thing for her child. She placed her baby with a couple in Christian ministry then went on to graduate high school and is currently married and attending college. "She has no regrets," Patsy says.

The Lighthouse also helped a twelve-year-old. Raped, then tossed out like refuse, this young woman attempted suicide before deciding to give The Lighthouse program a try.

"We witnessed a tremendous healing in the life of this young mother," Patsy says. "She gave her child for adoption. These results are wonderful and the whole purpose behind The Lighthouse."

Patsy and her husband Allen live as houseparents at the home. Her staff of volunteers currently consists of a nurse practitioner, who is overseen by a doctor, as well as experts in social services, counseling, childbirth, parenting, education, and job training. The Lighthouse has grown enough to offer salary to some of its staff. Lighthouse Ministries is operated through donations and fund-raisers.

Patsy would like to purchase one or more transitional homes. Though most women and their babies leave The Lighthouse upon being discharged from the hospital, it is the goal of the ministry to provide continued services for those who are not eligible for HUD (government housing) due to their age, criminal record, or other mitigating circumstances that prevent state and federal help. A home of this nature will offer an opportunity for these young women to live on their own, with their babies, yet still be under the covering of Lighthouse Ministries until they finish school, find jobs, and can support themselves.

Of all abortions only 1% occur because of rape or incest.[1]

While Bridegway and The Lighthouse help women, especially the young, through their pregnancies, many other women find many other forms of help for their specific, individual needs. In the following stories you'll read about other needs women faced, and where and how they found the help that met those needs.

The Miracle Baby, Anna,* and More

*by Marcia Samuels**
as told to Dianne E. Butts

Many women in our rural setting came to our pregnancy center for material needs: diapers, maternity clothes, baby clothes, and furniture, all of which were provided for free. I would ask them if they had a personal relationship with Jesus Christ. So many of them would just start weeping. They had grown up in religious homes, and they knew about God and hell and many things, but they didn't know they could have a personal relationship with Jesus Christ. This gave us many opportunities to help these precious ladies know Christ.

Not all the clients who came to the center were in a crisis pregnancy or were an abortion risk. One married girl who came in wanted so badly to be pregnant. Her lack of getting pregnant was her crisis. We prayed that God would open her womb. She did get pregnant, and she would stop in to see me. We called her child "the miracle baby."

We had other visitors at the center, too. I remember one man who came to us. I really can't remember what first brought him to our doors. There wasn't a wife or girlfriend. Nor was there a pregnancy involved. Still, he came in and we talked. He shared that he was an alcoholic, and I challenged him about his drinking. He came back to talk many times. Today he works at a local store and when he sees me, he always speaks to me. Recently his comments sound as if he's going to church now.

I too learned a lot while working at the center. I remember one young lady who called. She was pregnant and thinking of getting an abortion. I was very concerned, so I talked to her at length. I was very focused on trying to save her child from abortion. Finally she cried, "You don't care about me! You just care about my baby!"

Her words shocked me, but she was right.

I told her, "I am so sorry. I do care about you. Will you please forgive me?" I had to humble myself, and that was hard. But it turned out that admitting my wrong and asking for her forgiveness really opened up doors. She came into the center later. She'd made the decision to carry her child, and we were able to help her as she did carry to term.

And then there was Anna.* Hispanic. Catholic. And pregnant. She already had five children, and I sensed she was stretched to the limit. Anna asked about abortion. We talked about it, and Anna decided against it.

After her baby was born, she continued to stop by the pregnancy center and we would sit and talk. One day she told me one of her sons was having trouble in school. Other children were giving him a hard time, so we prayed for her son. Things got better for him.

"I've never had an 'Anglo' friend," Anna told me. I think that's really what Anna needed during that stressful time in her life—a friend.

*About 14% of recent births
to women 15 to 44 years of age
in 2002 were unwanted at the time of conception.* [2]

Turning Point

by Helena Grant

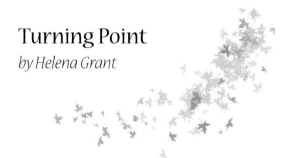

I came to Turning Point Pregnancy Care Center over a year ago when I heard of their need for volunteers. My heart was touched since I was once in those same shoes. At that time, I received so much blessing from others. Maybe this was my opportunity to bless someone in return, to give back to God something of what He had given me.

One day as I was sitting at my desk in the center a phone call came in. A young lady was in a desperate situation. She was pregnant with nowhere to go and no one to help her. Her mother was very angry with her for getting pregnant, and her voice sounded very much like mine had such a long time ago.

I could hear her crying out, so I told her not to worry and to come to the center to fill out some papers. I promised I would do whatever I could to help her. She came with another friend who was also pregnant, but although her friend was also single, her parents were allowing her to stay at home with them.

I listened to her story. She was with an abusive man. He thought of her as his wife even though they had not gone to the courts or the church to get married. He was a nonpracticing Muslim. She had been raised as a Catholic, though her family only attended church on holidays.

I asked her what her own beliefs were and she was not sure. She said her friend came from a born-again, Christian belief system, and that she had given herself to God when she was small and did that mean anything? Before she left to return to a motel where her mother was keeping her for safety reasons, we prayed asking God to guide her and provide for her.

Over the next hour, we both tried calling different shelters only to find all of them filled to capacity. So she left with my cell phone number. We stayed in touch even though I only worked one day with her at the center.

I went home and told my husband the story. We prayed together. His heart was also softened, as were my two daughters'. They all asked for this young girl to come and stay with us. We have two extra bedrooms.

I asked the center's director if this would be okay. She said I should do what my heart was telling me to do.

Without further thought, I took her in. She was not a problem to have in our house. She was grateful and helpful, something I had not found in many other people who I had helped in the past. We found her a job, an apartment, and she attended my church every Sunday. I counseled her at home, and we found a therapist who would take her without charging a large fee. We also found her a car so that she would have the freedom to come and go as she needed.

Among recent births:

64% occurred within marriage,

14% within cohabiting unions,

21% to women who were neither married nor cohabiting. [3]

We attended birthing classes together, and all was going smoothly until she decided to allow her baby's father to come back on the scene. When the time came for her baby to be born, she asked me to be there because we had grown so close. She had become like a daughter to me. Her mother did not like this, and many times gave me her opinion about it and ask me to abandon her daughter. But I could not.

My client had a baby girl! What a thrill it was for me to hold this precious child. The delivery was complicated, but she pulled through. Her mother was concerned because the baby's father was right back in her life. This didn't last for long, however, because he quickly became abusive again. He was heavily into drugs and alcohol and was not able to manage his temper. Even though he claimed to have given his life to Christ, his drug addiction was more than he could handle, and so she ended the relationship.

The new mom is now once again in a new home with a good job. And since then, she has not gone back to her old ways or to her parents for help. She actually lives very close to us, which makes us very happy.

She has a new man in her life, too, who loves her daughter and her daughter loves him. They plan to get married soon, and I pray that they will do well. They both still attend my church and have a great future ahead of them.

Would I do it all over again? Yes! I will always thank God that He brought this young girl to me.

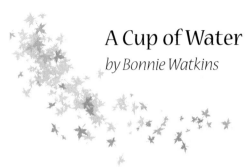

A Cup of Water

by Bonnie Watkins

My heart raced with excitement as I drove to the address of my first PAL, Lydia.* PALs, a program of a LifeCare Pregnancy Center, stands for "Partners in Affirming Life." As a PAL, I'm connected with pregnant clients and serve them in many ways. I might drive them to doctor's appointments, pray with them, shop with them, go through parenting or adoption workbooks with them, or even go through birth with them.

Smiling as big as her belly, Lydia met me at the door of her tiny efficiency apartment. She began to unravel her story. "I've been on my own since I was fourteen," she said. "My mother abandoned me. I quit school and got by as best I could, staying sometimes with distant relatives, other times with friends. I took what babysitting and cleaning jobs I could. When I turned sixteen, I got a job in a restaurant. That's where I met Frank.* Now I'm pregnant."

Here we were. We talked for hours. Lydia amazed me with her maturity and resourcefulness. One of my main ways to help Lydia was to drive her to the free clinic for her prenatal visits since she didn't have a car.

Frank, who was initially supportive, got spooked by the upcoming responsibilities. Like so many others in Lydia's life, he left her.

Then Lydia asked me, "Would you be my labor coach?"

I told her I'd be honored.

So, two pillows in hand, we attended childbirth classes together at the pregnancy center. We learned about relaxation, stages of labor, breastfeeding, and baby care.

124

Early one morning while it was still dark, my phone rang. "It's time," Lydia breathed quickly into the phone.

We walked the hospital halls together for twelve hours. When a contraction came, Lydia stopped and rested her head against the wall, and I rubbed her back and coached her through it. The nurses pretty much left us alone and so we walked alone, but together, until it was time for delivery.

Jeremy,* my first "adopted" son, entered the world screaming and with a full head of dark hair. Lydia prayed aloud, "Thank you, Lord, for this son. I will always love him."

Thinking to myself that Lydia was showing me maturity again, I added my own prayer: "Help Lydia to always take care of her baby, Lord. Thanks for the gift of allowing me to be present at one of Your miracles."

Our training as PALs instructed us to stick with the girls and their babies for about one to two months as they needed us, and then to move on so they wouldn't become dependent on us and so we could be available to accept a new PAL. With Lydia, I hung around for about six months, still driving her and Jeremy to the clinic for follow-up and well-baby visits. I rubbed the knot on his little leg when he got his first shots and it pained me as much as my own sons' had.

The next client who requested a PAL had very different needs. Cary's* primary request was help moving since her mother lived with her and was available to see her through birth. However, the mother had psychiatric problems and often had explosive episodes of anger that terrified both Cary and me. I spent hours just listening to her talk about her relationship with her mother. For Cary, I packed, cleaned, lined shelves, hung curtains, and rocked little Tierra* after she got home from the hospital to the new apartment. I began to have a "feel" for how long the clients needed me after the births, and Cary separated from me by fewer calls much earlier than Lydia had. With Cary as with Lydia, I felt that I had not been the spiritual mentor I would have like to have been. Time was always short. It seemed we rushed from practical thing to practical thing. Many times when I returned, I wondered why I hadn't just taken a few moments to pray. Often I just forgot spiritual matters in the midst of so many physical needs.

Tina,* sixteen, came along with a very different set of circumstances. At first, Tina's parents were very upset with her and told her they'd have nothing to do with her and this pregnancy. But, being a close-knit Christian family, her mother and father changed their minds and invited her to live with them after she had stayed with various relatives. My role in this pregnancy was limited after her parents became very supportive. I did meet with her and we started to go through the center's workbooks with very practical questions about parenting, finances, and adoption. Although we started strong, Tina and I only got through about two lessons.

Like Cary, Tina did not request me to be her coach since she had her mom. And since Tina stopped doing the lessons and I was unable to motivate her to continue, we didn't even get to the sections on spiritual growth.

Lord, I prayed, *"I wonder if I'm doing anything valuable here. Often I just seem to be a taxi service and garage sale shopper. Let me know whether You want me here or not.*

Later, I pushed open the hospital room door. Tina was holding her little bundle all wrapped up and peeking out of a blue blanket. "So, tell me all about it," I said. "What's his name? How much did he weigh? When was he born?"

She beamed. "Jonathan,* which means Gift of God. Seven pounds and two ounces. Two days ago at 10:00 p.m."

"You're kidding!" I said. "That's not only my birthday, but the exact hour I was born."

Okay, God, I thought, silently laughing to myself. *I get it. You've sent me a clear message that although I may not be moving mountains, You must want me to stay here for whatever good I'm doing.* Maybe by filling physical needs, I was filling spiritual needs that I didn't see. I was reminded of the Bible verse that says, "If you give even a cup of cold water to one of the least of my followers, you will surely be rewarded" (Matthew 10:42, NLT).

Betsy* came along next. At twenty-two, she was my first PAL mom who wasn't a teenager. Already a strong Christian, we spent more time together just hanging out and talking than I had spent with any of the other girls, which seemed to be her need. She invited me to be her coach. "Just in case my sister can't get here from South America," she said. Again, with pillows in hand, we attended childbirth classes at the center. Her sister did make it to the hospital and, along with another close friend, the three of us walked in and out of labor support for Betsy. Anthony* was born one hot August day, healthy and hearty, but after a long labor and eventual C-section. I spent many months seeing Betsy a couple of times a week to take groceries, do laundry, and clean.

Two more girls followed. One I met once and she never called back. I still pray for her and her baby. Another I called and we talked dozens of times on the phone, arranged meetings, but never met because she was sick throughout the pregnancy. I still pray for her too and call them PALs.

Teen mom Gisela* and baby Michael* followed. All of our talks and prayers were in the car outside her mother's apartment. Her mother was needy too and on several occasions drove up and talked with us.

Older mom Liz* needed a labor coach. She was my first PAL after having a heart attack a year earlier. I wondered if I would have the physical strength to assist her. God was very present with us through eight hours of back labor where I rolled a tennis ball on her back. Angelica* popped into the world quickly with prayers of thanksgiving.

Over twelve years in PALs, I have been the richer one. I have learned to serve more, pray more, trust more. And besides my two birth sons, I have eight more kids!

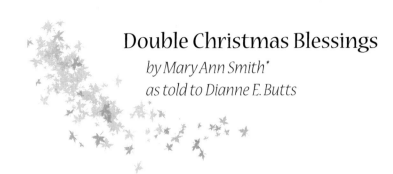

Double Christmas Blessings

by Mary Ann Smith*
as told to Dianne E. Butts

A number of years ago, before pregnancy centers had ultrasound equipment, I got a call from a student at the local university. She was pregnant and wanted an abortion. "My parents always said they would disown me if I got pregnant," she said.

I asked her to come in to the pregnancy center. She did, and we talked. "I just keep thinking of never seeing my family again, of no more Christmases together," she cried. She seemed so adamant about having an abortion so her family would never learn of this pregnancy, and yet she also seemed so conflicted about it.

"Why don't we schedule you for an ultrasound?" I suggested. I hoped the additional information provided by an ultrasound would help her in her decision. I knew a doctor in a city not too far away who did ultrasounds on his lunch hour, a kind service to women in need. She seemed skeptical about going.

"Well, let's do a pregnancy test to confirm you're pregnant," I suggested. She said she had already confirmed it and knew that she was, but she was willing to confirm it again with me.

We did the test. It showed negative.

She said the tests she had done at home were all positive.

"This is very strange," I said. "It's very rare to get a false positive. I truly don't know what's going on." She didn't either.

"The only way I know of that we can find out for sure if you're pregnant is with an ultrasound," I told her. She agreed. We scheduled the ultrasound and she made the drive.

128

When the doctor first saw it on the screen, he excitedly said, "Oh! We have two babies here!"

She came back to the pregnancy center to talk to me. "I could have gone through with an abortion of one," she said, "but not two."

We helped her through the pregnancy and beyond, and the next year at our annual pregnancy center's banquet there she was, pushing a double stroller . . . with her mother beside her. Her mother came over to me and thanked me over and over. "We thought we were doing the right thing, telling her we would disown her if she got pregnant. We thought it would keep her from behaving irresponsibly," she said. "Thank you so much for helping her. We're so grateful to have these two grandchildren . . . *and* our daughter in our lives!"

Resources

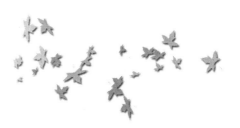

Need help in your unplanned pregnancy?
Find help here:
• The Heidi Group: http://www.heidigroup.org/
• "Directory of Shelters for Pregnant Women" listed by state at www.LifeCall.org, lifecall@aol.com, (800) 662-2678.
• Find a list of maternity homes at www.HiddenChoices.com.
• Assemblies of God Family Services Agency: http://www.agfamilyservices.org/, (800) 235-0652
• Option Line: http://www.optionline.org/ or 1-800-395-HELP (4357)

A Bible New Testament (with Psalms and Proverbs)
especially for women in a crisis pregnancy:
• *NIV Hope for the Future*, available from www.BiblicaDirect.com.

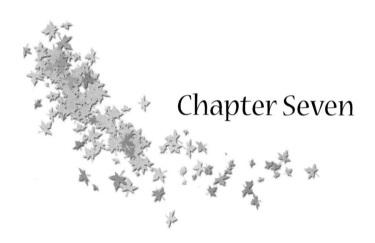

Chapter Seven

When a Woman Gives Her Child for Adoption

The LORD protects the simplehearted;
when I was in great need, he saved me.
PSALM 116:6

Sometimes giving a child for adoption is the most loving option.
Watch and listen as these women consider this difficult choice. See
how things turn out for them. And see how some become the waiting
arms that welcome a child and give him or her a home.

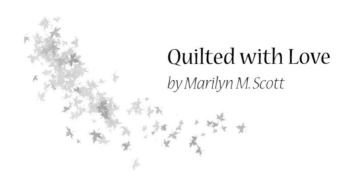

Quilted with Love

by Marilyn M. Scott

She was seventeen and angry. A pregnancy was *not* in her plans. She had made efforts not to become pregnant: she faithfully took her birth control pills and her boyfriend always used a condom. Despite their best efforts, the test read positive.

I sat across the desk from her. Her boyfriend sat in the waiting room. "What am I going to tell him?" she wondered out loud. She spoke her questions, yet didn't wait for my answers. It was as if she were asking her own conscience. Did she have to tell him? Maybe if she lied and said it was negative no one would ever have to know. Could she just go and have it "taken care of"?

I listened quietly, then began to ask questions to help her sort out her feelings and decisions. I told her about the baby growing inside of her.

"A baby? Is there actually a baby?" she asked. "Or is it like my health teacher says: just a clump of tissue?"

I showed her real pictures of a baby in the uterus at ten weeks gestation.

"Ten weeks?" She asked out loud, yet more to herself as she handled the pictures. Why hadn't she realized what was happening inside of her? Hands. Toes. Heartbeat. Brainwaves. She seemed amazed that this had been happening inside her without her even realizing.

I told her about families who would adopt her baby. Or if she wanted to, she could keep her child and parent. I told her what help was available to her.

She continued to answer and respond, but it looked like so much of what was being said was going in one ear and out the other. She repeated certain phrases: Post abortion syndrome. Possible medical problems. Parenting classes. Supplies. School. Adoption agencies and attorneys . . . She seemed to catch the main phrases, but I felt certain the details escaped her. She just stared at the two tiny lines on the pregnancy test.

Before we had started the test, I had told her, "Two lines represent a positive pregnancy test."

Two lines, her expression seemed to say. I imagined her thinking, *Oh why couldn't there have been only one?!*

"Can I pray with you," I asked.

"Okay," she answered. "I need all the help I can get."

After the prayer, I offered her a hug. And then I handed her a small, delicate handmade baby quilt. "This quilt was made by a senior citizen who wants you to know of God's love for both you and your baby," I told her. A small handwritten tag bore a Scripture verse and a prayer.

"I don't need the quilt," she said. "There isn't going to be a baby."

"Please keep it anyway," I told her. "You may use it to comfort yourself in times to come."

She took the blanket, and she and her boyfriend left.

I went home that evening with my heart heavy. I feared this young lady was making decisions that would haunt her for years to come—and would destroy her first child. I said many prayers for this client. I tried to contact her, but was unsuccessful. Between her job, school, and sports, she was never home.

A week later I was surprised when she entered my office. She shared with me what had happened the day of her scheduled abortion.

After she left my office, she headed to her car, unlocked the trunk, and tossed in the quilt. She didn't want her parents to see it. They would ask questions.

She made an appointment for the abortion. Her boyfriend would drive her to a city two hours away for the procedure. They would tell the clinic she was nineteen so her parents would not be notified. She'd been told she looked older than she was; this time she was counting on it.

A little lie to hide her age, she thought. One more lie piled upon the many others she had told in recent months. She lamented how things would have been different if she had not told that first lie to her parents about where they were going that evening. She never would have gotten pregnant.

She had traveled the road to the city many times, but for happy occasions like shopping trips with her mom, school outings, and church trips. But that day the road seemed long.

Neither she nor her boyfriend had much to say. Silence had become the norm in their relationship. Just when she didn't think she could endure the quiet any longer, a rumbling began at the back of the car. Her boyfriend said a curse word and pulled to the side of the road.

Great. A blown tire. He opened the trunk and pulled out the spare tire and tools to change it. She stood and watched. Not helping. Not speaking.

As he changed the tire, getting in and out of the trunk for the tools he needed, he pushed the small, delicate baby quilt out of the way several times. Each time his hands, now greasy and dirty, touched the small blanket, she cringed. Couldn't he see he was going to ruin it? Why wasn't he being more careful? Someone had made that especially for her and her baby!

When he finished, he heaved the blown tire into the trunk. She snatched the quilt just before the tire landed on it. She swaddled it to her chest. Tears streamed down her face.

He asked her what was wrong, but she couldn't answer. They got back into the car. She clutched the quilt, knowing he was probably wondering what he had done this time to upset her.

As they approached the next exit, she told him to take the off ramp. She told him she had changed her mind and couldn't go through with an abortion.

The trip home went quickly. Together they planned how to tell their parents. They tried to decide what was best for their child. Would they parent? Or would they choose one of the many couples waiting to parent their baby? They weren't sure, but they had time to decide and knew where to go for information on both options.

That small baby quilt had changed her life, she said. Now she wanted more information on adoption and wanted to ask questions about parenting.

At the end of our time together, she asked if she could give me a hug. I was usually the one asking that question!

I followed this client for the next six months. She delivered a beautiful baby boy whom she placed in the loving arms of two wonderful people who would be his new parents. She thanked me for the baby blanket and told me she had wrapped her baby boy in it at the hospital for the two days she got to spend with him. Now she sleeps with it and says she will treasure it always.

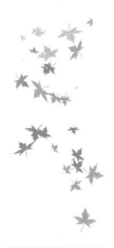

In 2002, about 2% of the adult population in the United States aged 18 to 44, or nearly two million persons, had adopted children. [1]

137

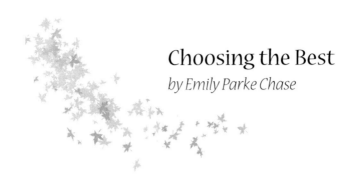

Choosing the Best

by Emily Parke Chase

She walked into my office at our local pregnancy center at age seventeen. She had never planned to get pregnant, but one night of sex changed everything. Now Elise* was pregnant and had a sexually transmitted disease as well. She felt like all her hopes and dreams had shattered and lay in a heap of shards at her feet. She didn't want to see this baby. She told me she just wanted someone—anyone—to take it away and place it in a home.

We began to meet regularly to talk about her plans for herself and her baby. When her parents kicked her out of their home, our pregnancy center found a local family who promised to care for her through the pregnancy.

One day, Elise arrived with news that a vague relative of hers in California wanted to adopt her child. The more Elise talked about the circumstances, the more concerned I became. "My cousin says he'll pay for all my medical expenses," she told me. "And I can live with his family for free during the whole pregnancy. He even has a job lined up for me."

"Elise, that sounds very generous." I said. "But what would happen if you changed your mind about the adoption and decided to keep the baby? I'm concerned you might feel pressured to go through with the adoption because he had already paid for all your expenses."

"Oh, it'll be okay," she replied. "He really wants the baby."

As I probed further, I discovered this cousin wasn't married to the woman with whom he lived. He already had several children by a prior relationship. To me, red flags fluttered everywhere like pennants at a ball game. But Elise didn't seem to think there were risks ahead of her. None of my concerns shook her confidence that everything would work out well.

"What about family reunions?" I asked. "Will you see this cousin at reunions?"

"Of course!" Elise said. "Our family gets together every year, so I'll get to see my baby then."

"Elise, do you think you'll ever want to marry and have kids in the future?"

"I hope so," she said.

"How do you think your child might feel seeing your new family and knowing that you placed him for adoption? Would your child wonder why he was placed for adoption but you kept your other children?"

"He'll understand," she said. Elise brushed aside my anxious thoughts as if she were sweeping crumbs off the table.

The day before Elise was to leave for California, she came to say good-bye.

Nothing I said seemed to diminish her determination. I talked with her again about God's love for her and His desire to walk with her through each step of her journey, but Elise hardly paid attention as she dreamed about her exciting future in California.

Elise left my office. I knew I'd done my best to help her think through her decision. Though her choice was not the one I thought best for her, I trusted God would watch over her. I called a team of people who pray regularly for me and told them, "Please pray for a young woman I've been talking with. She's making some difficult choices. She needs God's help."

They began praying around 4:00 p.m. that Friday afternoon.

One hour later Elise was packing her suitcase and preparing to say good-bye to the family who had taken her in. Suddenly, she walked out of her bedroom and into the kitchen where her temporary "mom" was fixing dinner. For the first time since her arrival, Elise burst into tears. Together, Elise and her foster mom reviewed her decision to leave. But this time Elise came to a different conclusion. She decided to stay.

That Sunday, Elise went to church with her foster family. With tears streaming down her face, she asked God's Son to erase her past choices, take control of her life, and guide her in the future.

Elise still planned to place her child for adoption. She chose a Christian adoption agency and began meeting with their counselor. But when their counselor tried to encourage her to look at profiles of adoptive families, Elise refused to become involved in the decision.

Elise continued to meet with me regularly as well. One day I asked, "Elise, would you want the mother of your child to work outside the home or remain at home with the baby?"

"I want her to be a stay-at-home mom," Elise said. "If she's just going to put this child in day care, why, I could do that myself! The whole point is that I want her to do what I can't: stay home and raise the baby."

"You could tell the adoption worker that is important to you."

"You mean I can choose a family where the mom intends to stay at home?" she asked.

"Sure! Would you like to have your child grow up in the city or in the country?"

"I have a choice?"

"Elise, that's what those family profiles are all about. They help you make key decisions that will impact not only your child's future but your life as well."

Before long Elise was studying the prospective adoptive parent's files. She picked out a family where the parents' hair was the same color as her own. "That way my child looks like he belongs," she explained. She chose a family who raised horses, "because I love to ride," she said.

She made other important choices, too. She opted to complete her GED course work and reestablished a healthier relationship with her parents.

 140

When Elise first came to our center, she was alone and without hope. She didn't even want to see her own baby. But by the end of her pregnancy, she had found a new church family, friends, renewed hope for her future, and a home for her child. She made good choices and chose the best.

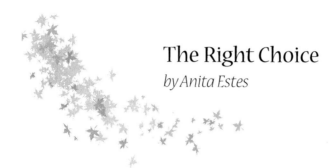

The Right Choice

by Anita Estes

When I volunteered to help with the Mentoring Moms program sponsored by New Paltz Pregnancy Support Center in New York, my first task was to call the women who had signed up to participate. I listened as the phone rang and rang in my ear. Finally, someone answered. "Is Natasha* there?" I asked, waiting expectantly.

"This is Natasha," a woman answered. A slight accent colored her voice.

"I was told you signed up for the Mentoring Moms program at the pregnancy center," I said. "I'm your volunteer mentor." We chatted a little and then arranged to meet at Natasha's apartment.

When I arrived, Natasha greeted me with a warm, broad smile that belied her deep needs. Natasha's one room basement apartment had no stove, only a lonely hot plate stuck in the corner of a makeshift kitchen, and a sink so small you could barely fill a glass of water. *Okay for a college student, but not a young mom*, I thought.

Natasha possessed a captivating beauty. We formed an immediate bond. I drove her to her Lamaze class and we talked.

At the hospital, the lessons flooded me with memories of my first sessions with my husband beside me. I wondered how Natasha felt having to practice with someone she just met, having a stranger fill in for a friend. Yet the lessons went well with me trying to model the breathing techniques. At the end of the session, Natasha asked, "Would you like to be my birth coach?"

I was stunned. How could I, a new acquaintance, share such an intimate experience? "Are you sure you want me?" I asked. Natasha nodded. "I never thought I'd need to do this again," I said, "but I'll give it a try." I not only became her mentor but her coach as well.

It was a crash course in mentoring since Natasha was my first case as a volunteer in the Moms program. Natasha was very needy, beyond what I expected. So I sought advice from one of the program's coordinators. I asked Rose* for guidance in helping Natasha. Rose's balanced approach guided me, and I leaned on her.

My first priority was to help move Natasha as her due date was approaching and her landlord wanted her out. Good apartments are scarce in a college town, so we searched together. I remember when we had to climb a flight of stairs that would challenge a mountain climber. Natasha did it in spike heels. I feared for her life, the baby's, and mine!

It turned out the arrangement for the apartment was one room in a messy apartment with three other guys! Natasha wanted to take it, but I coaxed her out of it. "You'll never make those stairs with a baby in hand," I told her.

But that left Natasha stranded. What could I do but take her in? The mentoring program never expected this from me, but I felt God was calling me to walk the extra mile. And I felt His grace to do it. Natasha had made a difficult choice to carry the child and not abort like many other college students. I wanted to support Natasha's choice and be the extended arms of the pregnancy center.

My family and I set her up in our enclosed porch in the back of the house and put her few belongings in storage, except for her books, which she loved. We had some difficult adjustments. Once again I consulted the program coordinator, Rose, to guide me. Natasha had grown up with an alcoholic father and mother, and she possessed few domestic skills. She didn't know how to cook or clean or do the laundry. Both the center and I tried to teach her.

But there were other problems. One day I came home from work at 5:00 and she hadn't gotten up yet. She told me she had trouble sleeping and later confessed she had frightening dreams. I stayed up nights talking and praying with her.

Although some people told me I had done enough, I still felt God wanted me to go a little further. I spoke to Natasha about Jesus and she listened. She told me she believed in God. In the evenings we prayed together for her circumstances and the baby.

The big day arrived three days after Christmas.

I called the pregnancy center for prayer then drove Natasha to the hospital. Natasha's labor was difficult; her level of pain unexpected. Natasha struggled to do the breathing. She asked for an epidural. It took the doctor five tries. At last he got it in.

Finally, Natasha gave birth to a beautiful seven-pound boy, Jacob.* She spent two days in the hospital before I brought her home.

After two weeks, Natasha moved into a nice apartment with another young woman and her child. The day I took her and Jacob there she said, "Let's be friends forever. Let's never lose contact."

I felt so touched. If it hadn't been for the Mentoring Moms program, I never would have met Natasha. I felt it a privilege to serve her and to be at the birth of her son.

But I knew what lay ahead. So I enlisted people from the pregnancy center and my church to help Natasha. I, along with the pregnancy center, had a baby shower at Natasha's new apartment. We provided her with everything she would need. Natasha felt overwhelmed with love and support and she

143

expressed her gratitude. It was wonderful. Afterwards, I, along with others at the pregnancy center, helped babysit while Natasha went to her college classes. But we didn't do it all. We wanted her to learn.

Even with all this help, Natasha encountered problems she'd never dealt with before. She had difficulty nursing the baby. She decided to use the bottle. She felt guilty and I told her that wasn't a problem, but it became one. One of the other volunteers told me Natasha stuck a bottle in Jacob's mouth every time he cried.

I communicated with Natasha almost every day. We discussed her struggles. Natasha mentioned adoption. Several times. I listened. I began to believe adoption might be the best solution, and so I discussed the idea with others at the pregnancy center. We prayed for Natasha and for God to guide her in making this decision.

One day Natasha phoned me. She was crying. She told me she couldn't handle being a mother. She asked me about adoption again. I advised her to consider it.

Natasha arranged a meeting with the pregnancy center director to discuss it. For over two months Natasha toyed with the idea but couldn't decide.

When the semester was over, Natasha returned to New York City and her friends. I thought it might work out, but after three months of desperately trying to mother the child, Natasha realized she just couldn't.

I spoke to her about the information she had received from the pregnancy center about adoption. "Only a terrible mother would do that!" Natasha insisted.

"No," I reprimanded her. "A terrible mother wouldn't care about the child. You care. Sometimes adoption is best. We, the center and I, support you in this decision."

Natasha consented to adoption. She sought an agency with open adoption, one in which the child would know his biological mother. She found one and after about two months, she received a call about an interested couple. Jacob was six-months old, and he could be the answer to a childless couple's prayers. The husband was a doctor. They lived in a beautiful home in one of the nicest cities in New York State.

Although she agreed to it, Natasha still struggled with the idea of adoption. She missed the appointment to sign the papers several times. But she finally she signed.

Jacob now lives with a couple who love him deeply. Natasha was invited to a welcoming party and she said everyone was so supportive. They gave Jacob all the love and attention she could ever want for him.

In my experience, adoption is a choice few women in crisis or unplanned pregnancies consider. They often misunderstand, I think. One girl told me it was heartless. It's not. Although adoption was difficult for Natasha, she did what was best for the baby. It took courage on her part to give Jacob to a loving family who could provide for him in a way she could not.

Because the New Paltz Pregnancy Center assisted Natasha through the Mentoring Moms program and also helped me learn skills to help Natasha through her pregnancy, birth, and eventual adoption, I considered this program so valuable that when the opportunity presented itself, I became the coordinator and ran it for two years.

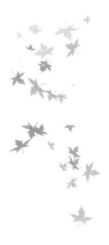

Never-married women continue to be the most likely group of women to relinquish an infant for adoption.

Prior to 1973, 20% of infants born to white never-married women were relinquished for adoption, compared with 1.3% from 1996 to 2002. [2]

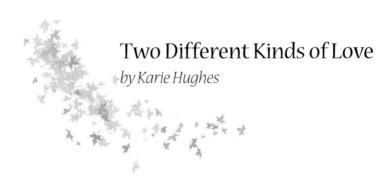

Two Different Kinds of Love

by Karie Hughes

I thought nothing really happened the night I went too far. I got up, left Kent's* home, and drove away thinking, *Oh my goodness. I'll never do that again!*

In the following days, the thought kept occurring to me: *Could I be pregnant?*

I decided to purchase a pregnancy kit at the store. In the privacy of my own bedroom, I took the test. A bright blue cross appeared. I was shocked. I really was pregnant!

This didn't fit into my life at all at this particular time. I had no money, time, or space in my small home. How would I care for this little life? I was already a twenty-eight year old single mom raising two children and recently divorced.

What if I have an abortion? I thought. *Then no one would ever know.*

I'd had an abortion at the age of fifteen. *Fifteen!* I struggled with the idea and had made the appointment at a local clinic believing it was "the easy way out" and "no one will know." Probably the biggest pressure I felt back then was the statement that an abortion would "let me get rid of the problem." I struggled for weeks before I made my choice. Then I went back to my high school with an imaginary mask on telling myself, "No one will know. Just go to class." But the choice of abortion is never the easy way out. The most important people know: Me. God.

And get rid of the problem? The baby is *never* the problem. The problem was me and my thinking. I wanted and longed for love, but I always settled for sex.

 146

I knew I could *not* have another abortion. Not this time. I was older. I knew what a baby looks like in the womb. Fully formed at eleven weeks. Heartbeat. Brainwaves.

Weeks went by. I was scared to tell people, but I knew I had to.

I will never, ever forget my friend, Janie, and her response. I envisioned a finger pointing at me while shaking her head back and forth saying, "I can't believe you!" But this is far from what happened.

"I'm pregnant," I said.

She picked me up and twirled me around and around. She was so excited that I was carrying a life.

I needed another option, though. I could not raise this child. A dear friend called after hearing I was pregnant. She had been the director of a crisis pregnancy center. She suggested I visit the crisis pregnancy center near me in Tempe, Arizona.

The counselor at the pregnancy center encouraged me to watch a video on adoption. I believed adoption was an unloving choice. *How can I give my baby away?* I thought. *I'll never know anything about this little life. Is this an unloving choice?*

I watched the video by myself. I was so moved by it that I took

52% of all abortions occur before the 9th week of pregnancy;

25% between the 9th and 10th weeks;

12% between the 11th and 12th weeks;

6% between the 13th and 15th weeks;

4% between the 16th and 20th weeks;

1% of all abortions (approx. 16,450 per year) occur after the 20th week of pregnancy. [3]

Where would the Lord lead me in my time of confusion? What am I to do? I thought it all over and made the appointment. This was the beginning of God's plan; He knew all along. (Journal, September 26, 1989)

About one-half of adoptive mothers are between ages 40 to 44 years of age (51%)

compared with 27% of mothers who have not adopted.

Conversely only 3% of mothers between ages 18 and 29 years of age are adoptive compared with 27% of biological mothers.[4]

notes while watching it a second time! *You mean I can choose the family? I can have contact through letters, pictures, and visits? It can be as open as I want it to be? Absolutely amazing!*

I cried. I knew right then this is what I would do. I would "place" (not "give") my baby with a loving family because I loved this baby.

Now Janie and I had something in common: She had adopted her daughter, Rachel. She was an adoptive mom, and I was on the journey of becoming a birth mom—the woman who would carry her baby for nine months and then place her child into a two-parent family home. Adoption wasn't the easy choice emotionally, but it was the right choice for me and this child. A loving choice. My loving choice.

On April 28, 1990, I delivered a beautiful healthy baby boy. Janie was there, helping me in the delivery room. When I handed Jonathon Aaron, a precious 7 lb. 5 oz. baby boy to the nurse, it was truly bittersweet. I felt deep joy knowing this baby would be in a loving home that I got to choose through open adoption.

It's just two different kinds of love: I gave this baby life; something the adoptive parents couldn't do. They would raise this child; something I couldn't do. Letting go isn't easy, but it's rewarding.

One month after Jonathon Aaron was born, the adoptive mom, Lyn, and I met at a restaurant. An older man walked past our table and admired the baby, sitting in his car-seat carrier. "Who's the mom?" the man asked.

Lyn and I remained silent. An uncomfortable pause lingered. Neither one of us knew who should speak. In a sensitive tone Lyn replied, "I'm the mom."

I leaned over and squeezed her hand. "Yep, she's the mom," I said.

The man walked away, probably bewildered because we took so long to respond. But Lyn and I just sat there smiling.

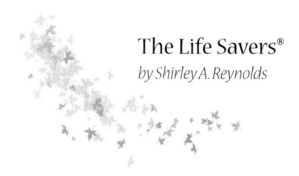

The Life Savers®

by Shirley A. Reynolds

I retreated to the quiet deck of our little mountain cabin. I flipped through the tattered pages of our photograph album. *Would Mandy* ever contact us?* The thought once again crept through my mind.

The memory of Mandy's dedication ceremony still brought tears. That was the last time I'd held her, but as I gazed at pictures from her adoptive parents, pictures of camping trips and school photos, holidays and her sister's hug, I knew there was no other choice my daughter, Sarah,* could have made. There was a picture of Mandy singing in church. *She's the spitting image of Sarah,* I thought.

I envisioned Mandy, dripping wet as she climbed out of a swimming pool. Her sister wrapped her arms around her waist and someone snapped a photo. As I viewed her adoptive grandpa giving her a "grandpappy" hug, a momentary sadness overtook my thoughts. Since my daughter had chosen an open adoption, communication between us and Mandy came through letters and pictures.

The decision Sarah made for the tiny infant she dedicated in a small hospital room was made out of love, a love God miraculously bestowed to a seventeen-year-old teenager. *Oh, but to only be able to hold a grandchild for a brief moment,* I thought. Letting her go was the toughest thing I've ever done as a grandma.

That dedication day I stood in the doorway of Sarah's private hospital room and watched as she cradled her tiny infant. I remember thinking, *My daughter, only seventeen-years-old, is a mother. Hard to comprehend.* I remembered the day Sarah came home from the family service center. She said she was going to talk to a counselor about options for her baby, but she had chosen to carry her baby full term. A picture, she said, was her turning point, along with a radio ad.

Our pastor arrived with the adoptive parents and their three-year-old daughter. Together, with my husband, Ken, we all gathered to dedicate little Mandy to God.

Ken held Mandy to his chest. He stared at her as if he was trying to etch her features forever into his memory while he prayed. When he handed Mandy to me, my tears soaked the blanket wrapped around her body. With trembling lips, I spoke; *"Oh little Mandy, we love you more than you know!"* Shaking, I placed her in the arms of my daughter. Sarah reached out and cuddled her new baby. She kissed her cheek and tilted her head up while she sang a song to Mandy. After a few words, she cried. With her arms quivering she handed her precious child to our pastor.

He spoke, and the room was absolutely quiet. Touching Mandy's face with oil, he prayed. "Little Mandy, I dedicate you in the name of the Father, the Son, and the Holy Spirit. May God bless you, and keep you in His care."

Weeping broke the silence. As Pastor placed Mandy into the waiting arms of her new adoptive mother, she too let her tears fall. Looking at Sarah with tears clouding her own eyes, she smiled at my daughter. Through her veiled joy, she seemed to convey sorrow for the young birth mother who was giving away her most prized possession.

Standing next to his wife, Mandy's adoptive father wrapped his arms around his new family. He also smiled at Sarah, as if to say, "Thank you."

When I looked at my daughter, I saw her empty arms. Tears streamed down her cheeks. *So many tears!*

Suddenly the little blond-haired, blue-eyed three-year-old daughter pulled away from her father and stepped in front of Sarah. In childlike sweetness, she looked into Sarah's eyes and placed her hands in her lap.

"Why are you crying?" she asked. "Do you want a Life Savers®? You know what? Life Savers® help you stop crying. My mommy said so." She squeezed something into Sarah's hand, and for a moment their hands entwined. A hint of laughter found its way into the grandparents and new parents.

Then a nurse, who had entered quietly, carried Mandy to the children's ward while Pastor and the adoptive family left the room.

Silent tears. Empty arms. Stillness. What should we have said? The tiny baby, who crept into our hearts in such a short period of time, was gone.

Sarah looked at me and her father and said, "She went to a special family, didn't she?"

"Definitely," her father said.

My wise daughter said, "I do believe that little sister was a confirmation. Maybe it was God's way of saying it's okay."

I saw Sarah's hand clenching the white peppermint Life Savers®. "Shall I throw that candy away?" I asked.

"No mom. I will keep this forever!" Sarah said. "It's a

promise. I will see her again someday. I know I will. For now, I'll say good-bye."

I gaze at pictures in the photo album. Mandy is now eighteen years old. *Wow. Where did the time go?* I keep thinking of the little three-year-old who was so touched with emotion for my daughter. From that chubby little hand a promise rose with hope.

Sarah is now a juvenile probation officer. She often tells her story to other young girls who are living stories so similar to hers.

When the road seemed hard to travel in past years, we have both looked at a package of Life Savers® and remembered.

There's a picture of eighteen-year-old Mandy on a horse, I thought. I compared her picture to one of Sarah's. I stared at the resemblance. *I do believe she has Sarah's brown eyes!*

Two months later, I saw that Mandy does indeed have the same brown eyes as Sarah. She and her family reunited with my daughter at our little cabin in the mountains. We rejoiced. It was a special miracle from God, our ultimate lifesaver. He did indeed replace ashes with beauty and mourning with gladness as Isaiah 60:3 says when He answered the prayers of this grandma.

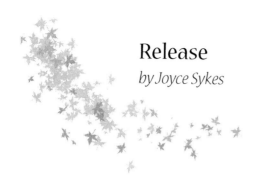

Release

by Joyce Sykes

December 20, 1970, I watched a social worker walk out the door with my beautiful three-day-old infant. I was sixteen years old. The previous five years leading up to that day had been pretty rocky.

When I was eleven, my mother passed away. My father remarried his first wife just a few months later. Angry, first at Mom for leaving, then at God for taking her, and now at Daddy and this new woman in our lives, I felt the tension build between my stepmother and me. She called me a whore and other horrible names.

Then I discovered my parents weren't my parents, they were, in fact, my grandparents. That completely rocked my world. My whole world was a lie, and I was devastated.

I longed to find someone to love and sought love from guys, not comprehending they were after one thing. The inevitable happened in March 1970 when after having sex with my boyfriend, I heard something speak to my heart: "You just got pregnant!" A few weeks later I missed my menstrual cycle. Then came the morning sickness. I was fifteen years old, terrified, and my boyfriend had already moved on. Instead of finding love, I was more alone than ever before.

When my stepmother realized something was happening, she made a doctor's appointment. On my sixteenth birthday I entered an examining room to hear the words I already knew: "You're pregnant." I was five months along, but had kept most people from knowing. I had already felt this innocent soul moving inside me.

My dad was heartbroken. My stepmother gloated. I had proved all her words true.

When we got home, Dad asked me, "Do you want an abortion?" In 1970 *Roe vs. Wade* was not yet, only backdoor procedures. But there was the question. What would my answer be? I longed for nothing more than this nightmare to end, but *no!* I knew in my heart that was not a choice. I had felt movement. I knew there was life. No matter how hard, I had to see this through to the end.

Dad seemed so relieved. But what now?

My stepmother would not allow a whore to remain in her home ruining her good name, so immediately a court proceeding declared me incorrigible and a ward of the state. I was packed up and moved to a maternity home in Durham, North Carolina.

College students did Bible studies with us. They did not look down on us, but shared the love of the Lord that they had found. Each had a relationship with Him like I had never seen, a relationship with a living and close Savior. They got excited as they felt the babies moving in us. Still, the image of being bad stayed with me for years, even long after I came to know the Lord Jesus Christ as my own Savior and came to know His forgiveness.

The time to deliver drew near. I wanted to go home for Christmas. Yet I had decisions to make. I didn't want this innocent life to suffer for my mistake. I could not give her a decent home. I was sixteen, barely in the 11th grade, and wondered if her father even remembered my name. Adoption was my only choice. I made my choice and waited.

Early on December 17, my labor pains started. A housemother took me to Duke Hospital where I was prepped for delivery and left alone in a room. My fear grew with each contraction. I gripped the railings until my hands cramped.

I was moved to Delivery. Mirrors hung all around. This was the last thing I wanted to see. I asked the nurse to please move the mirror. She snapped, *"Just close your eyes!"* I guessed she felt I was getting what I deserved. The doctor delivering my baby

 154

jumped up, slammed the mirror away, and let her have it for her insensitivity and judgmental attitude. His act of kindness stands out to this day.

Finally he told me, "It's a beautiful little girl!"

To the world she was the mistake of a bad girl, but this beautiful little one was mine. Allowed to give her a name temporarily, I chose Angela Mae because to me she was an innocent little angel and Mae was my mom's middle name. That was the only thing I had to offer, and I knew it would only be with her a short time. Her adoptive parents would choose her name.

Just three days passed before I had to release her. The social worker took her out of my arms and carried her to a place unknown to me. I left the maternity home with an ache that refused to be filled.

I made it home in time for Christmas, but I would only be there a few days before being moved to a foster home. The foster parents were stern, but they loved me and would not allow me to continue down my destructive path. Soon I met and fell in love with a neighbor's son. I stayed with my foster parents a year and a half until I graduated and married the following week.

My husband and I had a son. He was born just days from Angela's birthday. I watched him grow and celebrated each birthday, yet each year marked the passing of a birthday for the daughter I would not see. Decembers were rough.

My second daughter was born six years after Angela. My children made my memories less severe, yet the pain never left. I often wondered, *If I had one more child, would it make up for the one I betrayed by giving her away?*

The percentage of infants given for adoption has declined from 9% of those born before 1973 to 1% of those born between 1996 and 2002 or about 7,000 infants annually.[5]

I became an overprotective mom. I feared my daughter, Tammy, would walk the same path I had. When she was fifteen, I told her the truth. She was shocked, yet she immediately wanted to find her sister. I then told my son, Allen.

Also surprised, he asked, "You mean I'm not your oldest?" That made me smile. "Dad," he asked, "am I your oldest?"

Constantly I asked the Lord to protect my little one. *Send people to share Your love and grace with her,* I prayed. But I would not actively seek her. Did she know she was adopted? I remembered the tailspin I experienced when I learned the truth of my parentage. I couldn't take a chance of delivering that news. What if she was content with her life and did not want me in it? I had to trust my Lord with her life. If it was the Lord's will, He was more than able to bring us together.

Then one day at church, a woman gave her testimony of placing her daughter for adoption. She'd also had an abortion, yet she had such peace and joy. I talked with her, and she shared how the Lord brought her to a place of forgiving herself and allowing healing to come. Her story gave me hope where I'd had none before.

I began volunteering at a pro-life pregnancy center. To become a counselor, the center required me to complete an adoption workbook. Each painful lesson cleansed wounds bringing healing and great release to my spirit.

In late 2004, I registered with two online adoption reconnection groups. I wanted the door open if she came looking for me. In one website, you enter the information you have and anyone fitting that description comes up. However in North Carolina, adoptive parents can change the birth date and location. Had they change dates and places?

After work on March 7, 2005, I typed in the same information I always had. Except this time I made a major blunder: I mistakenly entered my son's birthday as the date of birth. Two new entries appeared. One said she was born in Durham and her mother was at the same maternity home where I had been. I remembered this infant, but this was not my child.

She had been so sick everyone thought she would die. My heart ached for the mother who probably thought her child had died and for the daughter whose mother would never check the adoption sites.

The second new entry listed the birth date as December 17. It was so close. The age of the birthmother: correct. The birth town: correct. Even the name Baby M could be correct. But she was using the name Melinda and the birth date of December 17. *Could this be her?* I wondered. Finally I closed down the computer and went to bed, all the time wondering about the date.

Early the next morning I kept thinking could they have changed . . . the . . . date? Oh my gosh.

My mind raced. I had entered the twentieth. That was not Angela's birth date; that was Allen's! Angela's was the seventeenth. I stood looking at my reflection in the mirror, toothpaste foaming at my mouth. What should I do next?

I went to work. At lunch I told my husband, "I think Angela is trying to find me!" We talked about my next step.

After work, I went to the website. I stared at the entry again noting the e-mail address. *What do I write?* Uncertain how much information to give about myself, I decided to simply ask questions. "If you don't mind," I e-mailed, "I would like to ask you some questions. Do you know which hospital you were born in? Do you know if your birthmom gave you the name Melinda? If so, I pray you find her. Like you, I'm looking for someone." I signed it, "Joy," clicked send, and waited.

Throughout the following day Tammy and I checked the new e-mail address. No mail. I arrived home from work to an empty house and raced to the computer. There was new mail.

I opened the message and began reading. My heart pounded. I had to calm down. I picked up the phone and called Tammy. I was crying so hard she thought I'd been in a wreck. When she realized I was trying to get out the words, "It's her. It's Angela," she raced to the house. We looked over the database entry together. Every bit of information was correct. I knew beyond any doubt. My daughter was found.

Now I had to reply. My hands shook. I realized she had only entered her data on March 3—just four days before I found it. I wrote a brief e-mail revealing all the information Melinda (a.k.a. Angela) shared was indeed the same as my own, except for one fact. Again I included the wrong date. I did not realize this until the next day. Oh what a mess this could make! I did not have a single doubt she was my daughter. But would she think I was taking her information and filling in the blanks?

Her reply was cautious. Melinda asked questions, which might be simple for most people to answer, but with my parentage, how would I answer? I could explain the date mix-up. But the other? I answered the questions, prayed the Lord would help her see the truth, and pressed send. Then waited again.

Friday, March 11, her answer came. Would she acknowledge me as her birthmom or reject me? Her words leapt off the screen: *"Yes, you are my birthmom."* I wept. My daughter, who was lost to me, the Lord had brought back into my life.

We spoke for the first time that evening. She told me I had made the right decision. She had a wonderful life with wonderful, loving parents. Only a week later I embraced the daughter whom I had not held in thirty-four years.

In the months that followed, we wrote almost every day and talked at least once a week. We got to know each other and realized how much alike we are. When friends see our pictures, they're amazed at the resemblance.

I can never make up for the time we did not share, but I learned she was a blessing to a childless couple and was blessed by their love for her. What seemed so tragic in my life blessed numerous people we've shared our lives with over the years.

Resources

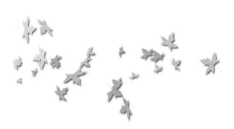

 Organizations:
Click "Adoption Organizations"
on the "Adoption Alternatives For Parenting"
on www.HiddenChoices.com, 1-877-488-9537
Bethany Christian Services:
http://www.bethany.org/

 Thoughtful article here:
"Adoption: Five Myths and Realities" on the
Presbyterians Pro-Life site here:
http://www.ppl.org/5myths.html

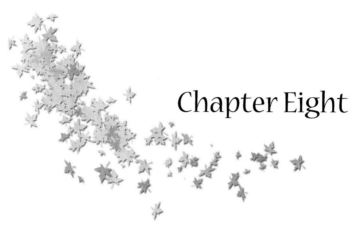

Chapter Eight

Who Are These People Who Help Women Find Options?

The Lord is gracious and righteous;
our God is full of compassion. . . .
Be at rest once more, O my soul,
for the Lord has been good to you.
PSALM 116:5,7

When facing an unplanned pregnancy, women, men, and whole families can find compassionate, nonjudgmental help at a pregnancy center. But just who will they meet there? Who are the people who run these centers and work in them? And how and why did these pregnancy centers get started?

In this chapter, you'll meet some women, men, and young people who staff pro-life pregnancy centers. You'll learn who they are and how they came to be there.

For some women (and men), their work has been borne out of their own unplanned pregnancies. Others have never experienced an unplanned pregnancy, but they have other motives for pitching in to offer compassionate help. Some, like Judy Sluppick and her husband, George, were influenced to become involved in this work by someone very special.

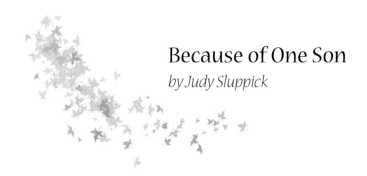

Because of One Son

by Judy Sluppick

I was an elementary school teacher, and never in my wildest dreams did I believe I would embark on another career. But in 1984 I found myself separated from my husband of many years. So I was living with my two sons, Darrell and Chip, in a lovely townhouse on the river, and we spent many happy days during that time.

My son, Chip, began attending an Assembly of God church. Before I knew it, he had been "saved." I wasn't sure what that meant, but I watched my youngest son do a complete turnaround in his life. Day after day, I saw there was something very different about him. He was a new creature in every way.

He talked to me about Jesus often. He told me that because of what Jesus, God's one and only Son, had done for us on the cross, we could be saved. This meant Jesus had taken the sins of anyone who looked to Him onto Himself and paid the penalty for those sins, and in exchange gave those who trusted in Him His righteousness—all in order to make us acceptable to God. Because of what God's one Son, Jesus, did, we can go into God's presence when we die and live with Him for eternity.

Chip invited me to his church and, after attending for a few weeks, he asked me one evening if I was ready to be saved by letting God come into my heart and life. Right there in our kitchen he led me in a simple prayer, and that's how he led me to the Lord. That is an awesome thing to happen to a mother. My life has never been the same since.

Along the way, Chip met some people who were involved in pro-life work and he heard about some training that was going to happen. It involved the opening of a crisis pregnancy center. Chip was very pro-life, and he suggested that I look into it and perhaps go to this training. I went and immediately knew this is where I belonged.

The doors for the new pregnancy center opened in 1989, and I began working as a volunteer peer counselor. Chip also helped the center with many of their endeavors.

Then in November of 1989, Chip moved to Shreveport, Louisiana, to begin attending a business college. He took his Harley-Davidson Sportster ™ with him. Unbeknownst to me, he had written to a motorcycling magazine, *American Iron*, and praised them for publishing such a clean magazine. He was not ashamed to keep it on his coffee table. He told them he was moving to Shreveport and if any Christian bikers would like to ride with him to let him know. Because he didn't yet have an address in Shreveport, he put my address and phone number down.

On January 9, 1990, Chip was in an accident on his Harley and died. Needless to say, I was devastated. We were tremendously close. Soon I began receiving letters and phone calls from people who were responding to Chip's article in the magazine, and I had the unfortunate job of telling them that my son had been killed.

One of the calls was from a man named George Sluppick. We talked for hours on that first call, and then talked on many days after that. I began looking forward to getting up in the morning and going to teach my third-graders. After many hours of phone calls, exchanging pictures in the mail, sending each other videotapes, and a few visits, George and I married on October 6, 1990. George was brought into my life because of my son, Chip. George rides a Harley-Davidson ™, and I love to ride with him.

163

In 1995 I became the Director of the Women's Resource Center in Natchitoches, Louisiana.

I'm now retired, but while I directed the center, George was such a huge part of the work we did there. I supposed he was our biggest supporter. He not only encouraged me but brought me lunch every day, helped with newsletters, moved furniture, ran errands, and more. At one fund-raiser banquet, George was one of our speakers. He spoke especially to grandparents because they are not often recognized as having grandchildren they've never met because that child had been aborted.

Many people may find it hard to believe that a Harley riding guy like my husband can be so pro-life, but he is. George has a talk show on our local radio station, and he often speaks for the unborn and encourages support for the center.

Although working as the executive director of the pregnancy center was challenging, I felt honored God placed me in that position. I often had the opportunity when counseling young women to tell them about my son, Chip, and that I am here because of this one son. It is also a perfect opportunity to tell them something more I learned from Chip: that God's grace and mercy can get you through anything.

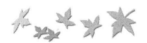

About 2,300 Christian pregnancy centers operate in the United States.[1]

Harley Grandpa

by George Sluppick

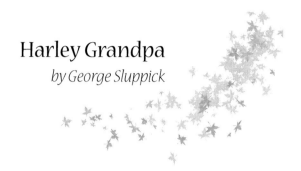

In 1990 I was living in Memphis, Tennessee, working as a credit manager for a pharmaceutical firm. Marriage number two had gone south, and I was raising a bunch of teenagers by myself. I had finally gotten back in church and had started producing live musical events on famous Beale Street and leading Bible studies at a local liquor store.

I rode a 1980 Harley-Davidson Roadster™, and one day I picked up a copy of the biker's magazine, *American Iron*, and found it to be a decent, clean publication. A letter to the editor from a fellow in Natchitoches, Louisiana, said he wanted to correspond with other Christian bikers. The letter said his name was "The Chipster." I wrote him a letter, not really expecting to hear back from him. A couple weeks later, I got a call from his mother thanking me for my letter but informing me that Chip had been killed on his Harley Sportster the day before that magazine hit the stands.

She and I talked for nearly three hours that first call. After that, we talked on the phone and wrote to each other a lot. I finally met her in person Easter week of 1990. After I left her, I firmly felt the Lord was saying, "Son, you picked the first two. I'm picking this one for you." Two weeks later, over the phone, at 2:30 in the morning, I asked her to marry me.

I soon learned there were some addendums to our marriage contract. First, I had to accept Judy's son Darrell, which was easy. I and all my children already loved him dearly.

Second, I had to accept the family pooch, believe it or not named "Scooter." That didn't take much. He was soon listening to me most of the time.

And finally, I was to give Judy as much time as necessary to work at the crisis pregnancy center. She had been working there as a volunteer since they opened their doors.

The "I Dos" came six months later. My Judy climbed on the back of my iron pony and we were off.

With Judy's work at the crisis pregnancy center, it didn't take long for some old feelings to surface. During my two combat tours in Vietnam, I saw many, many souls dead, maimed, and damaged in other ways. The children especially affected me. These little ones did not deserve to be part of a war nobody seemed to understand. I knew then that somehow I would have to do something that preserved life instead of being part of a system that destroyed it. Because of my wife's work, my long remembered desire became real involvement.

I decided not to be content with giving Judy her space to work at the crisis pregnancy center. I could do more. And I did. Maybe it was just bringing the gals some lunch or moving furniture or taking things to the storeroom. I built a pass-through with a privacy door for the ladies to place their pregnancy tests. I was their handyman and courier. I organized a fund-raiser concert and booked a comic, a ventriloquist, a preacher, and a ton of music. I even wrote a poem to be read during the concert for all the grandparents who are often left out of the picture.

"From Grandpa"
by George Sluppick
Just wanted to say, "Hi,"
And I love you very, very much.
I never got to know you,
What you looked like, who you were.
I never knew if I was to build you a dollhouse
Or take you fishing.
I didn't get the chance to take that picture of
You in your tutu . . .

Or was it shoulder pads?
Would it have been GI Joe or Barbie at Christmas?
Would the ribbons have been pink or blue?
At your wedding, I didn't get to
Figure out which side I was supposed to sit on.
Grandma and I wonder, Do we count you as a grandchild?
Would you have blessed us with great-grandchildren?
No matter. I'll see you soon enough.
You're with Jesus now.
Just wanted to say, "Hi,"
And I love you very, very much.

The ladies at the center had no problem if I came blasting up on my Harley Ultra Glide™ or later my Tour Glide™. One of the gals, Nikki, took a picture of my Tour Glide™ the day before she took off for Africa to minister to families of AIDS victims.

Sometime later I found out the executive director was stepping down. I took it upon myself to talk to one of the board members about my Judy and her qualifications. I must have said something right, for she ended up in the driver's seat.

The pregnancy center changed its name to the Women's Resource Center and moved into a beautiful old home. And I was there, even after a heart attack. I may not have been able to lift and tote, but I helped direct and unpack. I drew designs for the counseling rooms and helped set up the supply area. I could still run a water hose quite well for an old biker, and so I washed the outside of the building. I've been a speaker at our fund-raising banquets, and Judy and I usually worked together on her monthly newsletter. I checked in with them every day, and usually there was something to mail or pick up or take to the Goodwill® store.

I am now the news director and host of the morning call-in talk show on one of the local radio stations. My Judy has been on the show several times. We don't get many calls. Either she is a good guest with lots of information or people are too afraid to talk about the tough issues involved in the work at a pregnancy center.

The Bible tells us to minister to the least, and you can't get any more "least" than a tiny life in the womb. This is not just a lady's problem. New life blesses everybody. The taking of new life eventually hurts everybody. If I can do one thing that frees up one counselor to minister to one girl who changes her mind about having an abortion, then I've done what I'm supposed to do.

I have since been a feature writer on five articles for *American Iron* magazine, including one on the growing legion of Christian bikers. And how about that photograph Nikki took outside the crisis pregnancy center before she left for Africa? It was featured in *American Iron*. Thanks to our five great children, we now have four wonderful grandchildren and one great-granddaughter. Judy has since retired as director of the Women's Resource Center, but then went back as a volunteer. As for me, I too retired, but I'm still called upon once in a while to help out with the center's work. And I keep piling on the miles on my Harley™.

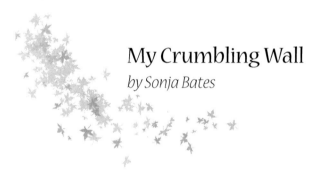

My Crumbling Wall

by Sonja Bates

I got pregnant when I was nineteen. The details of my story aren't that different from a million others, so there's no point in going into all of that. But I want to emphasize that I knew the difference between right and wrong. I was raised in the church. I went to church Sunday morning and Sunday evening as well as Wednesday night prayer meeting. I attended vacation Bible school every year until junior high and went to church camp a few times. When I had my abortion I had to override all of the standards that I had been raised with.

I regretted that abortion even before it was over, but in my mind there was no one to turn to for help. I never told my parents because I was afraid. My boyfriend told his parents, and they were completely in favor of abortion. In fact, they paid for the abortion of their first grandchild. I was filled with grief and anger, but there was no one to talk to about it.

Even though abortion is intentional, it is a pregnancy loss and women need to grieve. Suppressing the grief and struggling to keep your conscience quiet is utterly exhausting. The best you can do is weigh it down under denial. I remember my own rationalizations: unwed motherhood, parents' disapproval, financial fears . . . *Fear.*

I hated myself. Eventually I punished myself by aborting a second baby. I remained depressed and angry for years. I battled thoughts of suicide.

One Sunday in 1995 a man named George delivered a presentation in the church I was attending. George was the director of a pregnancy resource center. He told us about the center's services, which included a post-abortion Bible study. I couldn't believe it. I thanked God for the pastor who had such insight to bring George in and let him speak.

I was married to a very kind man who loves me to this day. We had a smart, healthy eight-year-old daughter, and I was a few months into maternity leave after the birth of our beautiful baby boy. I should have been happy, but I was a mess.

I had been deeply depressed for years, but I did my level best to hide that from everyone. At thirty-five years old I was worn out from trying to ignore all the pain and grief. I was ready to deconstruct my wall of denial. I wanted to learn to trust God and other people. When George showed up at our church, my wall was already crumbling and I was ready for help.

I attended that post-abortion Bible study with four other women. It started the grieving process, and I began to heal. When I finished the study, I knew I wanted to tell people the

169

truth about abortion and help other women find the peace and healing I had found. I now do that by teaching a post-abortion Bible study called *SaveOne* through the church I attend and through the San Bernardino, California, Pregnancy Resource Center.

Abortion hurts women and men. We are right to fight for the unborn, but we must also share Christ's love with the millions of men and women who have already experienced the pain of abortion. They need to hear that there's hope and healing in Jesus Christ. We can create an atmosphere of trust in the church and communicate to post-abortive men and women that it's safe to share their pain and grief with us. We can help replace their mourning with joy in healing and forgiveness.

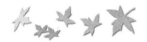

Care Net reports it has a network of more than 1,100 pregnancy center affiliates.[2]

My Mental File

by Kelly J. Stigliano

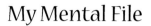

I was thirteen in 1973 when abortion was legalized. While attending our county fair in Ohio, my friend and I walked through the various mobile vans with displays hawking the owners' wares, pet projects, or issues. Most offered freebie giveaways and my friend and I didn't miss a single one.

We stepped up into one van and began looking at the photos and brochures. One in particular caught my eye. "A trash can full of dolls?" I asked. I looked closer. Those weren't dolls. I asked a few questions and left that van with handfuls of literature and my first understanding of what abortion is. *That's so wrong,* I thought, mentally filing that picture away.

Five years later, in 1978, I was unmarried and pregnant. Because of that mental file started in 1973, abortion didn't cross my mind. I married, had a beautiful baby girl, and sixteen months later had an adorable baby boy. It was tough but oh so worth it.

Then in 1982, when I was twenty-two years old, I prepared to make a hushed and hasty escape from my abusive husband and become a single mother of two toddlers. Two months passed with no menstrual period. An older woman at work suggested I get a "D&C." I knew what she meant. Facts from those old brochures shot through my mind:

> **"A baby's heart begins to beat
> at 22 days after conception."[3]**

> **"All biological indicators suggest unborn children are
> capable of feeling pain by at least 20 weeks."[4]**

171

I was torn. The thought of supporting my two children on my secretarial salary was daunting. The thought of having another baby, missing work, getting day care, and "catching up" financially was overwhelming. I decided to dismiss my conscience and follow my coworker's advice.

I called a women's services clinic, was told they did abortions, and planned to schedule one following my initial visit. But after two conflicting pregnancy tests, I left the clinic in tears. Two weeks later my period started. Although I didn't have an abortion, the guilt of deciding to abort lasted until Jesus healed my heart.

In 1986 I came to know Jesus as my personal Savior. I married a wonderful Christian man who loved my children as his own. We moved to Rochester, New York, and I was asked if I wanted to help at a crisis pregnancy center.

"Yes," I said. "I'd love to volunteer, but my kids are little and I'm not sure I have time." I was given an option that worked for everyone. After training, I became a weekend phone counselor. The center's phones were forwarded to my house one weekend per month. During that time I was on call around the clock. I loved this! In a season of my life that required me to be a full-time mother to my own little unexpected blessings, I could still help with a cause that was very near and dear to my heart. I totally got it. I understood the fear of being unmarried and pregnant, of telling parents the news, of being in an abusive relationship and thinking you're pregnant, of having made the agonizing decision to abort—even knowing it was wrong—and the ensuing guilt. Most importantly I understood that when everything looks hopeless, the decision to give birth and either parent or develop an adoption plan for the baby is all bearable with Jesus' help and guidance.

Late one night the phone rang, and I sprang out of bed. On the other end of the phone was an African American woman about my age. She had three children and was confirmed pregnant, but thought she'd had a miscarriage after having passed a "tiny pink thing." I checked my books, told her it sounded like a miscarriage, and suggested she get to the hospital right away. I made an appointment for her at our pregnancy center and later learned she had indeed miscarried. But "a tiny pink thing" kept going through my mind. *An African American woman lost a pink baby,* I thought. *We are all the same until God stretches that last layer of skin over us! How beautiful.*

Another time the phone rang late at night and I answered to hear loud crying. A young Asian college student, schooling in America, lamented the fact that she was pregnant and wanted an abortion. I told her we could help her sort out all of her options. I tried to set an appointment for her. "You don't understand," she cried. "Where I come from I have to be a virgin; I can't be pregnant! My parents will know I'm not pure!"

I assured her that her parents loved her and would be upset but would surely help her.

"No," she insisted. "I have to be a virgin! I can't be pregnant! You don't understand!"

She made an appointment at the center, but in my heart I knew she wouldn't keep it. A long night of tears and prayers followed at my house.

We now live in Florida, and in 2006 I was asked to be on a steering committee to help bring a new crisis pregnancy center to our county. The thought of being involved with this work again thrilled me and I accepted. In 2007 we met to discuss plans and funding options. By winter of 2008 funding had begun. It has been a whirlwind ever since.

My husband and I both volunteer at the center. My husband talks with the men who come in with their wives, girlfriends, and daughters. The new center is open now, in Clay County, just three miles from our home. We volunteer each week. We are blessed to help serve the more than one hundred men and women each year who previously had to travel to another county for pregnancy-related services.

Providing accurate information on all the choices to our clients establishes a complete mental file of information that helps them make good decisions for their lives.

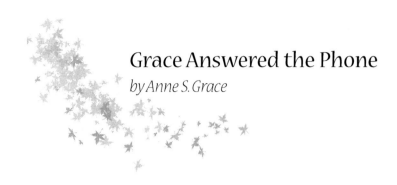

Grace Answered the Phone

by Anne S. Grace

When the phone rang that afternoon at the Woodbridge, Virginia, Birthright office where I volunteered as a counselor in the early 1980s, the lady calling had a strange question. "Is it possible to get pregnant after having a tubal ligation?" she asked.

"Yes, it most definitely is possible," I replied. "I know because it happened to me several years ago." She explained that she'd had a tubal ligation nine years earlier, but now she had missed her monthly period and wondered if she could be pregnant.

Following the birth of our third daughter in 1970, I had the tubal ligation performed. It is a form of sterilization that ties the fallopian tubes into a horseshoe shape and then cuts out two and a half inches of the tubes. Usually the severed parts shrink away from each other. Occasionally they touch and grow back together.

When our third daughter was thirteen months old, I, too, missed my period and recognized the disruption of my regular pattern. After an examination, we learned I was indeed pregnant. Following the birth of this child, a son, I had the operation performed a second time. However my doctor told me, "The procedure was done perfectly the first time. There were no mistakes."

With this in mind, I counseled the woman, "You can come to our Birthright office for a free pregnancy test, or you can go to your own OB/GYN doctor, whichever you prefer. But please see your doctor right away. Don't put it off."

At Birthright, we gave pregnancy tests (this was before the home tests became available), and talked with women who wanted information about adoption or abortion. When talking about abortion, we talked about abortion procedures, risks, and so forth. The only thing we wouldn't do was refer her to a doctor for an abortion or help her obtain one. We loaned car seats through our Kids in Safety Seats (KISS) program, collected kits for newborns with kimonos, receiving blankets, diapers, etc., and responded to daily phone calls. Each counselor wore a lapel pin of two petite feet, an exact replica of a baby's feet at ten weeks in the womb.

Each time I went to work, I wondered about the outcome of that lady's situation. Several months passed. Then one day while I was working, I answered the phone and it was she.

"I wanted to call and thank you," she said. "I did go to my doctor and found out I had a tubal pregnancy. Had I not called you for information, and had I not gone to my doctor, my tube could have ruptured and I could have died. Thank you for saving my life."

When I think of her calling our Birthright office and of me answering the phone with a personal example and knowledge of her situation, I thank God for His grace as He intervenes in our lives!

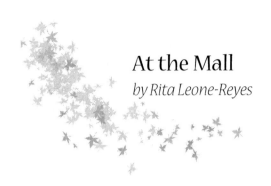

At the Mall

by Rita Leone-Reyes

I was a chubby, ethnic kid in elementary school with big hair and a strict family. I got teased all the time, and I had self-esteem issues for as long as I can remember.

I came to Christ at the age of ten, went to Catholic School, and I always liked boys. My first kiss was in the first grade with Tommy, the boy next door. Boys teased me a lot, and my mother told me that's what boys do when they like you. My dad was mean, so there had to be something to that.

I didn't date a lot in high school because I wasn't allowed to. When I was allowed to have my first date, I remember my dad went out to my date's car and checked his odometer. Dad wanted to make sure we stayed within a three-mile radius of the house. I was mortified! After that I never really encouraged boys to come to the house. I certainly didn't want them to meet my dad!

I went to an all-girls high school. I'm certain that was part of my father's strategic plan to keep me focused on my studies. I graduated with honors and without a boyfriend, so I guess it worked. After high school, I went to Drexel University for a year, but Drexel turned out to be harder than I ever imagined. I left Drexel to go to the community college and took a job at the Echelon Mall and there I met the man my parents would consider their worst nightmare.

I was committed to abstinence until marriage. My virginity was very important to me, so there was no way I was going to sleep with this man. However, I wanted this man to like me. And I thought "messing around" was really okay as long as I wasn't

176

"doing it." I was safe, right? My friends were all having sex. I was nineteen, and I could handle myself.

I started dating My-Parents'-Worst-Nightmare. He was twenty-six. And turns out he was expecting more than I ever wanted to give. On our first date he took me to a motel. I was incensed. Who did he think he was?! I didn't even know this guy! That should have been a red flag. I didn't get out of the car.

His response? "This was a test. And you passed." He was impressed with my virtue? Interesting.

We continued to date, and he continued to pressure me for sex. That should have been red flag number two. I didn't yet know that if your boyfriend (or, for guys, girlfriend) can't honor "No," then they can't honor you.

I kept dating him. I was in love with the thought of being in love. He was in a band. He really wanted me. I thought I was in control. Even God was whispering to my heart and mind about getting out of this relationship. I ignored Him . . . and the red flags.

My parents were getting more and more upset about him being in my life. He had no real job. He had no education. He had little motivation. He put up with them, but he frequently told me to quit listening to them. They didn't know who I really was, he said. They didn't understand our relationship. I didn't yet know that when someone starts to alienate you from your other relationships, that is a sign they are controlling. That is the beginning of abuse. I stopped going out with other friends. I stopped talking with my mom. He was the focus of my life. Even the Lord took a backseat. That should have been red flag number three.

What was it about this guy that pulled me away from everything I knew and loved? He was meeting a need in my life to be accepted and loved.

There came a point in our relationship when sex was all he would talk about. He wasn't going to take "no" anymore. I still thought I could control the pressure, but my objections fell on deaf ears. One day, on a date, he took from me what I had no intention of giving him. I was date-raped. It was the worst moment of my life.

I ran from his apartment. He lived near the Echelon Mall, so I ran there. I was bleeding terribly. I wasn't sure if it was because he forced himself on me or because it was my first time.

Can you believe there was a Christian ministry in that mall? The mall was owned by a Christian, and he believed shoppers should have a place to go and pray, and so there was this ministry office. I ran to it hoping to talk to someone, hoping to use the phone to call a rape crisis center, hoping to use the bathroom to clean up. But when I got there, the ministry office was gated shut. The mall was open, but the ministry was closed.

There I stood, locked out of that Christian ministry. I felt I had ruined my walk with the Lord and now I was on the outside looking in. I so longed to be in, but I felt locked out of His presence. And I thought this was all my fault.

At that moment, I hated my boyfriend. I hated him for hurting me and betraying me. But I hated myself more. What a fool I was. I had let God down. I had let my family down. I had let myself down. I had lost something I could never get back. It was done.

When I got home that night, while everyone was sleeping, I raced out to the trash and buried my bloodied pants. My mother could never find the evidence of what I had done.

Fear, guilt, and shame kept me in that relationship with him, now a sexual relationship. In six months, I was pregnant.

Of course he was ready to offer me his money for a quick abortion. His sister was also pregnant and she was getting an abortion. Maybe we could have it done together, he suggested.

His sister had her abortion and in less than a year was pregnant again, had her baby, and married the guy.

Nine months later I had my son and never looked back. My son is twenty-one years old today and I am so proud of him.

In 1996 with the help of my parents, we started a crisis pregnancy center. A few years later, our pregnancy center was approached by a representative of the Echelon Mall asking if we would put a pregnancy center inside the same ministry I had run to in that same mall. There was no way we could afford the mall's rent. But that ministry said, "You take the place for one or two nights a week and do your pregnancy tests." So we got the space for free.

And boy did we start to see girls come in like crazy. We were safe. They didn't have to lie to their parents about where they were going. They could just say, "Mom, I'm going to the mall," and they could stop in to see us if they needed help.

Later, we received a grant for an ultrasound machine, but our location in the mall was upstairs and for various other reasons it simply wouldn't work for that. So, as much as it broke my heart, we had to move our pregnancy center.

Then a few years ago we were approached by another pregnancy center forty-five minutes from our office. They asked if we would take over their center. We made the drive to check it out and discovered their location was old and dingy. The walls were cracked. It needed a lot of work. Plus, the lease was up.

But there was a brand-new mall in the area, with a Macy's, JCPenney's, and Sears. We checked into it, and not only was the space perfect for an ultrasound and all we needed, the lease was actually *less*. We've now been open at that location for two years.

I am thrilled to be back in a mall. It's as if God said, "You have to close your mall location, but you're not finished." Where I once was shut out from the Christians and the ministry that I desperately needed, I now have a place open for other girls and women who need us so much.

Heartbeat International reports it has over 1,100 affiliated pregnancy centers, medical clinics, maternity homes, adoptions agencies, and abortion recovery programs in forty-eight countries.[5]

You read her story, "Release," in Chapter 7. Now see what happened when Joyce Sykes wanted to volunteer to help others facing an unplanned pregnancy like she had.

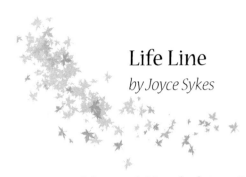

Life Line

by Joyce Sykes

I entered the cozy lobby of Life Line Crisis Pregnancy Center. The receptionist smiled and informed Michelle,* the director, that the prospective new counselor had arrived. Anxiously, I looked around at the multiple doors guessing some would be the counseling rooms where I might someday affect the lives of people facing an unplanned pregnancy. Little did I know how behind the closed door directly in front of me my own life would be affected in the weeks to come.

Michelle stepped into the lobby, smiled, and extended her hand. My first impression: this woman could be a friend for life. Her quiet nature reassured me, allowing me to relax a little. I followed her to her office.

The picture Michelle painted of the work performed in this little office became clearer as she spoke, putting me at ease. The painting was so vivid and inviting I knew I wanted to be a part of the work here.

But secret thoughts flew in the back of my mind. *If only this crisis pregnancy center had been here when—*

I forced my thoughts back to the conversation at hand. "What brought you to Life Line?" Michelle asked.

"While my children were in school, I was secretary and a teacher's aide at our small Christian school. But they've graduated, and I wanted to volunteer somewhere. A friend at church suggested Life Line."

"Great," Michelle said. "I feel we make a difference in our client's lives and their precious little ones." As I sat listening to her enthusiasm, I could feel a stirring in my spirit. Maybe my friend at church was right that the Lord was guiding me here.

Michelle stopped midsentence. "I sense there's more going on here than what you've shared. Do you want to talk about it?"

Shocked and amazed at her discernment, my tears began flowing. "I had a daughter when I was sixteen and gave her up." Shame once more welled up from a deep crevice of my heart. I could no longer look at her. She knew my horrible secret.

Michelle quickly moved to the sofa beside me and wrapped comforting arms around my shoulders. This simple act of kindness overwhelmed me, and deep, gut-wrenching sobs tore loose from my heart and lips. It had been twenty-six years since the social worker walked out the door with my three-day-old daughter. Only my closest friends knew this secret. I knew God had forgiven me. But the reality was I had never forgiven myself. A true mother would never have given her child away.

After several minutes, my heart began calming. Sheepishly, I glanced up. Amazingly there was no look of disgust, only the gentle smile of a woman who was not condemning me for my past failures.

My story is the same as many other young girls: looking for love and acceptance, a guy looking for something else, and the rest was history. By the time I realized I was pregnant, he had moved on. And in 1970, only bad girls did things like this. No one talked about it, much less kept the baby.

I was barely sixteen when my daughter was born. I had no home, no way to support myself or a child. My stepmother had me sent to a maternity home, then after my daughter was born, a foster home. I wanted more for my daughter than I could possibly give her. I wanted her to have a mom and a dad and the thought of this innocent child suffering because of my failures horrified me then and even on this day.

"Joyce, you will be a great asset at Life Line. You'll understand what these girls are going through because you've been there. But," Michelle said, "I require one thing. I want you to work through our adoption-healing workbook." She paused to see my reaction.

"Why?" I asked, taking a deep, ragged breath.

"For so long, you have hidden this wound. It's time. You need healing."

I knew her words were true. Forgiveness had come years earlier as I surrendered my life to the Lord, but situations around me constantly stirred old memories bringing bouts of depression. Even as I spoke with Michelle, the pain was still raw. Willingly, and yet terrified, I nodded my agreement.

With the book in hand that night, I settled down and began reading the material. Questions came, bringing with them long forgotten events that were difficult to think about much less put down on paper. Rejection. Desertion. Terror and fear. These emotions still felt overwhelming all these years later. The recollection of my father's pained expression when he realized the truth and the gleam of smugness on my stepmother's face.

Step-by-step, lesson by lesson, Michelle and I dug into the past. Each week the probing questions delved deeper into the untold shame and pain. Yet each week, a gratefulness rose in my heart for this ministry. How different my life and emotional history might have been if it had been available in 1970. Each session the wound was opened. Bit by bit my spirit gained immunity to the poison that had been hidden so long.

I was taking little steps toward freedom and healing.

Memories of the few acts of concern shown during this dark time in my life came to mind, overshadowing the negative for the first time in my life: a doctor who cared, college students who came to the maternity home and shared how the Lord loved each of us. These forgotten pictures became glimpses of the Lord's love and concern for me even then.

I accepted the reality I had made the right choice for my precious child. I had looked past what I wanted and made the best choice for this innocent one.

That adoption-healing workbook didn't change my past, but it did allow me the healing that changed how I looked at it. I had made a mistake and paid dearly for it. But the Lord had forgiven me, and most of all I had finally forgiven myself. The decision to let my little one go was the decision of love.

I went on to help numerous other women, men, and families through my volunteer work at Life Line. I still grieved for my little one, prayed for her, but left her in the hands of the Lord. He was with her. If He saw fit to bring us back together, this healing had prepared me for it in a way nothing else could. In time, He did bring us into each other's life in a miraculous and wonderful way. How grateful I am for organizations like Life Line. Such ministries had been unheard of years earlier, yet all these years later it could help bring me healing, hope, and restoration. And now I'm helping others find the same.

It's All About Me

by Connie Ambrecht

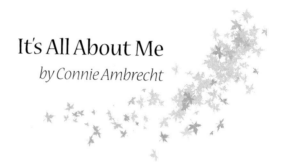

When I first entered the lobby at a pregnancy care center, I never imagined my life would change. I began my first evening of volunteering, and it seemed benign enough. No dramatic scenes unfolded. No shouting matches took place. No unhappy visitors made accusations. Instead, I saw young women, nervous and unsure about their futures, seeking support in welcoming strangers. As they opened their hearts to me, I became their sounding board. It did not take years of fond memories with them to win their confidence. I was the one person willing to listen to their struggle and advise them in this unsure time.

When I first applied to volunteer, my thought was, "I'm sure I can help them. My ultrasound skills should be useful." After all, the center had a sonographer listed on their list of needs that they were praying for. "I'll be helping them out," I thought. But after several weeks of playing phone tag with the executive director at the center, I began to feel that they must have filled that particular need with someone else.

I didn't imagine the executive director at a nonprofit community outreach could be so busy. She was. Extremely busy. Along with every volunteer and staff member. After I spent time at the pregnancy center, I realized just how difficult it is to find dependable volunteers with a strong commitment to the center.

After a few encounters with the young women who entered the pregnancy center's door and conversations with other volunteers and staff, I began to understand what I was doing was less about these troubled women and more about my walk with God. I'm learning it's not about what I can bring to the center; it's about what He can do in my life through the center and the women I meet there. It's about how I need to grow. It's about how He reveals Himself to *me* through each situation I see.

In most settings it can be presumptuous or offensive to think "it's all about me." However, I can see now that my walk with Jesus *is* all about me. When I try to help others, God really shows Himself to me and I grow. I see His hand evident in my life. He takes my shortcomings and turns them into fruit. He turns my preconceived notions into gentleness, my harshness into self-control, my judgments into patience, my criticisms into love and kindness.

Had I foreseen all He had planned for me when I set foot in the pregnancy care center, fear may have frozen my feet. But I'm glad I volunteer. It's so worth it.

When it comes to our relationships with God, it's okay to say, "It's all about *me!*"

"Too Many to Declare"
Dedicated to the volunteers and staff
at pregnancy care centers.
by Connie Ambrecht

How could I have known when I first
came through the door,
How my life would be changed forevermore.

I'll give my time. I hope they'll be blessed.
It was after my training that came the first test.

What do I say? I long to be truly heard.
Out of my heart comes the truth, the truth of God's Word.

How could I have known as I met each one,
I would see glory; I'd see His Son.

How could I have known, it almost seems strange,
How my life would be touched; there would be change . . .

Too many to declare, not one can recount,
The things you've done Lord, generous in amount.

The wonder of Him is seen in each face,
God's love is shown to all who enter this place.

Immeasurably more than we could think or ask.
With Him in the lead, we can accomplish the task.

185

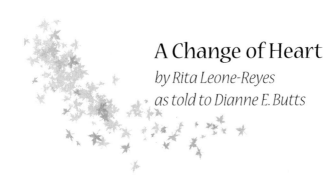

A Change of Heart

by Rita Leone-Reyes
as told to Dianne E. Butts

It was two doors down from a church—the doctor's office that provided abortions. Pro-lifers, which included some people from the church, had picketed this doctor's office. Many in the community had prayed he would have a change of heart about performing abortions. But he kept offering his services—first to anyone seeking an abortion, then later only to his own patients. We wanted to offer these same women hope and other alternatives. So we decided to open a pro-life pregnancy center directly across the street.

It was a time when many pregnancy centers were installing ultrasound machines. We wanted an ultrasound, but the laws require that we have a physician to oversee our program. We would require the doctor overseeing our program to never perform any abortions—even in his private practice. But in New Jersey, with 80% of private OB/GYN doctors performing abortions, how were we going to find such a doctor?

I was the founding director of this new pregnancy center. I attended a conference to learn all I could about how to run a center like ours. At that conference, an OB/GYN gave a presentation and told his story:

He had approached a Florida pregnancy center as a business venture. He wanted to get their patients as referrals. But his visit with them took an unexpected turn. After this Jewish doctor formed a relationship with the Christian workers in the pregnancy center, he came to believe in and accept Jesus as Messiah.

This man saw the need pregnancy centers had to be connected to doctors. His vision was to start an association that would link physicians to pregnancy centers all across the nation. Physicians would benefit by being able to expand revenue by getting patients referred to them, and they would be able to bill Medicaid. Pregnancy centers would benefit by having physicians on staff to oversee the ultrasound programs they wanted to implement.

This was the very help I needed! I believed this man could help me find the doctor I needed to oversee our ultrasound program in New Jersey. So after he finished speaking that day, I went looking for him. When I finally caught up with him, I told him my situation. "I need a doctor for my center," I told him. In my mind I wanted, and was praying for, a good-looking, young, male, pro-life, Christian doctor.

"I've contacted some, but none will talk to me because I'm just a pregnancy center director," I told him. He told me he had a directory of physicians on a CD that he would use to find a doctor in New Jersey. He promised he would be in touch.

It was only a couple days after I arrived back home following the convention that he called. "I've found a physician for you," he said.

"Who is it?" I asked.

"Well, his office is on, um, Gan-tower?" he said.

"Do you mean Ganttown Road?" I asked. "That's the street we're on! What's his name?"

He told me the doctor's name.

"That's the abortionist across the street!" I told him. I couldn't believe it. Then I asked, "He's actually interested in talking to me?"

"Yes," he said.

"I asked the Lord for a young, good-looking, pro-life Christian and you find me the old, pro-choice Jewish abortionist across the street?!" I asked, incredulous.

"Will you meet with him?" he asked.

I got my back up. As far as I was concerned, this man had blood on his hands. I wanted to scream, *Are you kidding*?!

"If I come to New Jersey to talk to this man," he asked, "will you come with me and talk with him?"

An opportunity to meet this doctor and talk with him personally about his work? I agreed.

When I met with these two physicians, the first thing the physician across the street did was begin to explain why he wanted to work with me and the pregnancy center. He explained that he was a *mohel*, a doctor who performs ritual Jewish circumcisions. He said when he held those little babies in his arms, babies that he had delivered, he couldn't help but wonder what had happened to the babies he had not delivered. Where were they now? He didn't want to do abortions anymore.

I told him, "If you work with us, you can't ever do another abortion."

He said, "I don't want to."

I asked, "When you have a patient who wants an abortion, what are you going to do?"

He said, "Send them across the street to you."

I was convinced. He wanted to stop doing abortions. We put all of that in writing. He signed on the dotted line.

He worked with us for about five years overseeing our ultrasound program and even appeared on our ministry videos to tell his story until he had health challenges and retired. At that time, we found ourselves back in the same position: needing another doctor to oversee our ultrasound program. We had another doctor approach us. He, too, had been performing abortions. He, too, wanted to stop. He saw us as his opportunity to stop performing abortions, and we gave him that opportunity.

In my mind and heart, I knew on my own I would *never* have worked with that first physician. But God changed my mind and heart. After all, He reminded me, we *had* named the pregnancy center "Choices of the Heart." I am awed by what man would throw away that God is able to use for good and His glory.

Resources

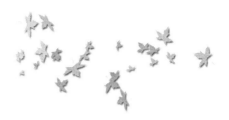

You can find caring people nearest you throughout the United States as well as in many other nations around the world here:
• Option Line: http://www.optionline.org/ or 1-800-395-HELP (4357)
• Heartbeat International/Our Initiatives/Global Advancement: http://www.heartbeatinternational.org/our-initiatives/global-advancement
United Kingdom: www.lifeuk.org, info@lifecharity.org.uk
United Kingdom: www.prolife.org.uk
Philippines: www.prolife.org.ph
Australia: www.prolife.org.au

In Ed's* story, "A Father After All," in chapter 5, Ed told us about his daughter who struggled with addiction while she was pregnant. If you're in a similar situation, have other special circumstances, or received a troubling prenatal diagnosis for your baby, you can find help from medical professionals here:
• American Association of Pro-Life Obstetricians and Gynecologists: http://www.aaplog.org/, 339 River Avenue, Holland, MI 49423, (616)546-2639.
• Pro-Life Maternal-Fetal Medicine: http://www.prolifemfm.org/
• Perinatal Hospice: www.perinatalhospice.org
• Choices Medical Clinic: http://www.choicesmc.org/pages/pregnant/perinatal.php, 538 S. Bleckley, Wichita, KS 67218, (800)879-7451.

Resources

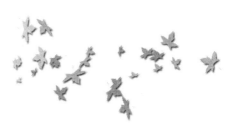

For those who receive a troubling prenatal diagnosis, find peer groups for encouragement here:

• Health Awareness: Prenatal Diagnosis: http://www.angelfire.com/ca/numberslady/.
Carry to Term With a Negative Prenatal Diagnosis: http://carrytoterm.org/.

• Strings of Pearls: Offering Hope for the Journey: http://www.stringofpearlsonline.org/.

Book:

A Gift of Time: Continuing Your Pregnancy When Your Baby's Life Is Expected to Be Brief by Amy Kuebelbeck and Deborah L. Davis, Ph.D. (Johns Hopkins University Press, 2010).

Chapter Nine

Reaching Out, Helping People, and Preventing Unplanned Pregnancy

How can I repay the LORD for all his goodness to me?
I will lift up the cup of salvation and call on the name of the LORD.
PSALM 116:12-13

The needs and heartaches of women, men, and whole families surprised by an unplanned pregnancy are as many and varied as they are. The staff and volunteers of pregnancy resources centers, also known as crisis pregnancy centers, offer a wide and equally varied menu of services and resources—many of them free. Besides pregnancy tests and counseling with a peer counselor like you've read about in so many stories in this book, many pregnancy centers are now staffed by medical professionals and offer services such as testing for sexually transmitted diseases right in their facilities.

Other pregnancy centers reach out into their communities with presentations and classes aimed as much at prevention of unplanned pregnancy as helping women and men in them.

The wide variety of help that can be found in and through these centers may surprise you. Hear the stories of how some centers are impacting individual lives, whole communities, and beyond.

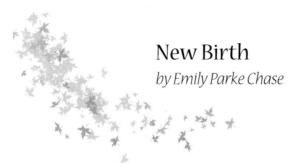

New Birth

by Emily Parke Chase

After an elder in her church sexually abused her as a child, Yolanda* became sexually promiscuous herself. She floated in and out of several abusive relationships. She took heavy doses of medication for depression. When she walked into our pregnancy center seeking help, Yolanda desperately desired to get her life in order. She wanted God to make her pure again.

Over the next months, I met regularly with Yolanda. I challenged her to make a list of the qualities she really wanted in a strong relationship. I told her only Jesus Christ could meet *all* her expectations, and we talked about how He might do so. I studied the Bible with her and she was willing to pray with me.

Time after time she would try to break off the relationship with her current boyfriend. Again and again she would return to him, yearning for the physical intimacy that made her feel loved.

Yolanda slipped out of my life, and I didn't hear anything more from her for over a year. Then the following letter arrived.

> Dear Emily,
>
> This year has been a year of new beginnings for me. In December, I prayed for three things: more faith, renewing of my mind, and for a final answer regarding my relationship with my boyfriend.
>
> In the late spring, God made it very clear to me that my relationship with my boyfriend was over. That relationship of two-and-a-half years was a painful one but I continued to push toward God,

194

and I know there were several people, especially you, who were praying for me.

Two weeks later, people from a Christian training institute came to my church. These men have recovered from drug and alcohol abuse and have given their lives to the Lord. One man sang a solo and gave his testimony of the goodness of the Lord. He entered the program seven years ago. In two years, the pastors sent him to Bible college. John* and I met at his pastor's house in June.

Soon after, John asked his pastor for permission to date me! Both his pastors approved, but they laid down the rules: We were not to officially start "dating" for six months nor could we hold hands!

John is everything I wrote on that list for you in one of our counseling sessions. He was who I was praying for, but I had to believe God could do it. John is a renewed virgin. He was delivered from a life of pornography and has not had a relationship with a woman, by choice, in seven years! He told me when we met that he was willing to wait for my healing from my previous relationship. I never knew someone like this existed, but he does and I am so grateful. I see that I am worth waiting for! God bless you, Yolanda.

PS: My medication has also decreased for the first time in three years.

A couple years have passed since then and, as it turned out, Yolanda didn't marry John. But she is still following Christ and pursuing her relationship with Him. She attends church regularly, loves singing in the choir, and still stops by to visit me occasionally. Yolanda didn't enter our doors seeking a pregnancy test, but a new birth took place nonetheless.

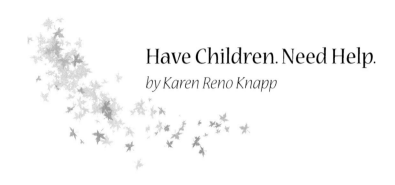

Have Children. Need Help.

by Karen Reno Knapp

No one remembers how Stacy* came to our Care Net pregnancy center in Hallstead, Pennsylvania, for her first visit. But we remember she was exhausted. With another child on the way, Stacy was overwhelmed with her two boys and a girl—all under the age of seven.

"I need help with my children," Stacy said. She was looking for suggestions for discipline and guidance. Stacy began meeting regularly with Cora Williams,* the director, and other Care Net counselors. She was especially interested in the parenting skills classes offered through the "Earn While You Learn" program and so she took that class.

Cora suggested Stacy take her children to story hour at the local library. "These experiences will help your children learn to listen to other adults besides their mother," Cora said. "And why don't you enroll your children in a Christian preschool? It would give you some personal time. Plus, it would teach your children about the Bible." Initially Stacy was hesitant about becoming involved with Christian ministries, but she began to see their value and began to trust input from the counselors at the Care Net center, so she enrolled her three older kids.

Her children heard Bible stories in preschool and began to bring home colored pictures representing the stories, which soon adorned the refrigerator. Then came the questions. Stacy's children began asking their mother about the people in the pictures. Often Stacy had no idea how to answer. She had attended church when she was younger, but that wasn't enough.

She needed more knowledge about the Bible. So Stacy began attending a local church along with her children.

Stacy was also invited to attend a Mom's Bible study and parenting class. The teacher was a Christian who said while raising her own family she'd "been down the same road" as those in the class. She understood the need for encouragement and guidance.

Stacy found the help she was seeking for her children and so much more, and it all began with a visit to a Care Net pregnancy center.

Campus Life 101

by Emily Parke Chase

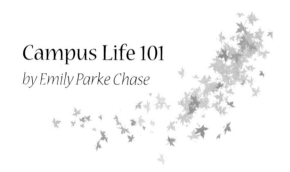

While in high school, Kendra* was date-raped. She didn't get pregnant, but she contracted genital herpes, a forever-reminder of a nightmare she wanted to forget. She felt dirty, used, and angry. Though her self-esteem plummeted, she managed to keep her grades up and move on to college.

Early in her first year on campus, Kendra volunteered to help with our pregnancy center's abstinence education program in local schools. She went with me to speak in individual classes, helped with skits, and shared her story of being hurt in a dating relationship. She hoped her testimony of pain would warn others and keep them from repeating her experience.

Now Kendra was sitting across from me in the coffee shop on campus. Staring down into her cup filled with coffee and twirling her spoon nervously, she said, "Emily, I'm pregnant."

My stomach twisted. I had grown to care for this gentle young woman with her elfin features and quiet smile. I had hoped that she was healing from her past, moving forward into a brighter future. I reached across the table and touched her hand. "Tell me about it."

In addition to the discomfort of morning sickness, Kendra was experiencing both regret and embarrassment. She had disappointed herself and let me down too. Her world was upside down, and she wasn't sure how to set it back on its axis.

"Kendra, does your boyfriend know about the pregnancy?"

"Yes, Brad's* fine with it and plans to stay with me. We plan to marry after we finish college."

"You are both freshmen. That means a wedding wouldn't be until several years from now."

"I know," Kendra replied. "We can't afford to marry. We'd lose our scholarships."

"Does your boyfriend know that you have herpes?"

"I told him before we had sex. It was hard, but I've been really up front with him. Because I was working with you and talking about my past with kids in public schools, I figured I needed to be honest with him too. When I think I am getting an outbreak of blisters, I tell him right away so he won't get infected."

"You know that herpes can be transmitted even when you haven't got an active outbreak."

"My doctor told me that too. Brad got tested and so far he's okay."

Over the next months, Kendra and I continued to meet. We talked about her plans to drop out of college for a semester. Then she'd pick up her courses again in the next term. I referred her to a pregnancy center near her hometown, but we kept in touch via cyberspace.

After she had the baby, Kendra returned to college. She sought me out and once again we met on campus. While I admired her baby boy, she caught me up on her life. She and Brad were still together. They were planning to move up the date for their wedding.

"After what happened to me in high school," Kendra confessed, "I wasn't certain how things with Brad would work out. Sure, God would forgive me and love me, but I wasn't sure I'd ever find a man who would accept me once he knew I had herpes. Brad and I have both committed our lives to Christ and placed our future in His hands. Brad knows there is a chance he will get herpes some day, but he's willing to deal with that."

Over ten years have passed since that conversation. Brad and Kendra did marry and now have two handsome boys. Brad continues to test negative for herpes.

Today, Kendra helps me in speaking to groups about sexual self-control. She still looks like a college student. The teens in the audience look at her and see someone who appears to be a typical Sunday-school girl and wonder what she could possibly know about what they are facing, but when she tells her story, they sit up and listen.

She tells the students, "I learned that trust, honesty, and love in a relationship become even more important when you have a disease like herpes. My husband Brad trusts me to tell him when I have an outbreak and I am honest with him. He loves me no matter what. If you have already had sex, don't lower your standards of what you are looking for in a relationship. Instead, raise your standards! There are others like Brad out there and they are worth waiting for."

Hope's Sexual Integrity Class

by JoAnn Valdez
as told to Dianne E. Butts

When I saw the curriculum for a sexual integrity class in 1998, I was so excited about it that I had the pregnancy center of which I'm the director, Hope Pregnancy Center in Trinidad, Colorado, purchase the materials. We watched for an opportunity to use it, but that didn't come about until the summer of 2009. A local Christian school, Holy Trinity Academy, heard about the program through a woman who volunteered at our center and liked the idea of reaching out to seventh- and eighth-graders to talk about sexual integrity. "We only have a few girls," they said. "Would you present the class to them during the summer?"

Fine! I thought. That summer class gave us an opportunity to get acquainted with the material.

In the fall, Holy Trinity Academy invited us to present the program to their high schoolers. Holy Trinity Academy started years ago as a Catholic school but later opened to other students. We had twenty-four students! About half were Catholic and half were Protestant Christians.

We met with the freshmen and sophomores in one class, and juniors and seniors in another class for eight weeks, which really gave us time to get to know each student. Together we worked our way through the two books and one video the program provided with the curriculum. We talked about integrity and self-respect. The curriculum guided us to talk about the whole person: intellectually, socially, physically, emotionally, and spiritually.

I love that this program allows us to talk with the students about God. We talked about sin and how it separates us from God. Then we talked about how we can be reconciled back to Him. We talked about how God wants to be involved in each individual's life, that He wants to be involved in writing each person's love story, and that we can trust Him with our relationships and future spouse.

I believe this sexual integrity class will have a lifelong impact on those twenty-four students and touch other lives beyond them. And we've been invited back to teach the class again in the fall.

Queen of Sexual Healing

by Patrice Egging

When I was the director of ABC Pregnancy Help Center in Pratt, Kansas, we tried to meet the physical, social, intellectual, emotional, and spiritual needs of each individual. Both men and women were welcomed and encouraged. During the initial consultation, one common thread seemed to appear time and again: that of sexual trauma or sexual abuse. Most clients did not see themselves as abuse victims. Most of them figured this type of experience was normal, that everyone went through the same thing.

Later, during training from Heartbeat International's Sexual Integrity Program, I discovered many women who seek help for a potential unplanned pregnancy have been sexually abused. I

One estimate is that over 70% of women who come to pregnancy resource centers have been sexually abused or traumatized. [1]

201

began to use the materials designed by Heartbeat at our center, and I can say that I saw some miracles. The videos, by Dr. Doug Weiss, *Steps to Sexual Health*, were my favorite resource from that program. They were designed as a peer-to-peer level of presentation, not a professional counseling session. I am not a trained psychologist, but these materials are terrific for helpers like me to use with the type of clients that typically come to a crisis pregnancy center. Any need for further professional help was always a referral situation. I showed these videos to men and women, young and old, in groups and with individuals.

Susie* was a typical client. She needed help with baby clothes and diapers. She lived with a boyfriend, not the father of her child. She was underemployed and sometimes unemployed. Susie was sexually abused in her early years by a family member. As an adult, she lived with an abusive man who nearly killed her, and she escaped with the help of a stranger. She met another abusive man who introduced her to methamphetamine. She was using crystal meth when she found she was pregnant. She stopped using and tried to get away from that man. In order to do so, she was "hiding out" and living with the current boyfriend. The mother of the boyfriend told her about our pregnancy center, and that's why she'd come in.

Susie watched literally every video we had in our resource center. The sexual integrity videos helped her reconsider her situation, and she left her boyfriend when he lied to her about his continued use of pornography. Susie decided that she wanted someone who loved her, respected her, and would not lie to her. She was also concerned about her daughter and did not want her in a situation that would be potentially dangerous.

Several years passed, and she recently began to attend a small church, deciding to let God have control of her life. It so happened that a young man was there that day who had basically led a similar life and was making a similar decision. They met, exchanged phone numbers, and are now married.

One older mother was referred to us for parenting issues concerning a teenage daughter. The initial conversation revealed that the mother had dealt with some childhood physical abuse, and at age fifteen she and a friend were both raped. Years had passed. She had experienced multiple sexual partners, prostitution, drug abuse, a failed marriage, and now a daughter in rebellion. When she watched these videos and worked through the exercises, I could see the "lights come on," a recognition that the trauma had initiated a series of behaviors as a way of coping with her pain. She realized that she did not need to stay in the pattern. A year or so after she had finished the videos I got a call from her. She was asking for information to help her niece. She was passing along what she had learned to help another person in pain.

Many times an individual would start the videos but not finish them. This bothered me a great deal. Then at a conference I got to meet Dr. Weiss, and I asked him about this situation. He told me there was no set way to use these videos: one could stand alone, any order is fine, and if a person were not married the last two could be optional. But what he told me next really had an impact on me. He said if God had called me to be involved in bringing healing to people who have been damaged sexually, that I was the "Queen of Sexual Healing" and that anything I did would be just fine. I was empowered!

In a group parenting class of ten women and men, seven had sexual trauma. I showed one of the *Steps to Sexual Health* videos to that group for an introduction to healing as part of the ten-class series. They learned if they had trauma as part of their past, it affects their parenting skills.

One woman saw only the first video, but it gave her answers to why she had stayed in a very abusive relationship. She saw a reasonable answer for something that she had previously blamed herself for. And she was hopeful to not make the same mistakes again.

Sometimes it was a volunteer who had a life changing experience. After viewing several videos, a volunteer came back from a weekend family reunion. During that visit, a name was mentioned, and flashbacks of her being date-raped came flooding into her mind. After that incident, her life choices had led her on a path of bad relationships and an eventual divorce. The videos had discussed this situation of suppressing memories and that they could be revived with a "trigger" stimulus. Because she had seen the videos, she was better prepared to begin to heal.

Many people have had some degree of trauma in their lives. Sexual trauma is especially harmful because it affects everything about you: how you think, how you behave, and even how you pray. I was so honored to be part of a process of healing for these clients. I pray that they continue to learn and grow toward healing and happiness.

I have since left as the director and the center now has a new name, location, leadership, goals, and programs. But I was privileged to be a part of the "birth" of ABC Pregnancy Help Center and honored to see the new Pratt Family Life Center continue to grow. They are building upon our foundation, continuing to serve the men and women in our Kansas community.

Georgia Red Clay

by John McNeal

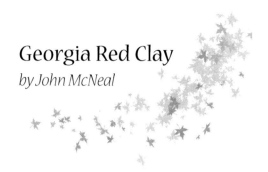

I spread out a large plastic drop cloth on the floor in the room filled with chairs but empty of any other person. The audience would be mostly youth groups this Wednesday night, bused in by their churches. As the students began to file in, I was awed that more than five hundred students, youth ministers, and chaperones had come.

Ann Gainey, director of the Gainesville Care Center, would introduce me. The Gainesville, Georgia, center's main focus was to help young women and men make a life-affirming choice for their unborn children and help prepare new mothers and fathers for their new lives as parents. I was there to speak to the students about abstinence in hopes that they would not need the Gainesville Care Center's other services.

Ann introduced me and I made my way to the front.

I asked for a couple of volunteers and found two girls close to the front who were willing to help. I then stood on the large piece of plastic. "Now reach in my bucket there," I directed them, "and get a good handful of that stuff."

They looked skeptical. "What is it?" they asked.

"A mixture of Georgia red clay," I told them. Georgia's red clay stains, making it nearly impossible to get out of anything it gets on. "Now begin to smear it all over my shirt," I instructed. I wore a white, long-sleeved button-down dress shirt.

They giggled as they spread the mixture all over my shirt. "This shirt represents my virginity," I told the audience. "That dirt represents sin and the other things that come along with sin." I began to name sexually transmitted diseases.

205

The girls suddenly stopped wiping the muck on me and stared at me. "It's only a representation!" I said.

Then I gave them something to clean their hands with—one, single regular restaurant napkin. They were really good about getting the muddy muck off their hands and out from under their fingernails. But they still had some left on their hands, so I asked two guys to come up and help them remove the rest of the mess. The guys couldn't help but get some of the Georgia red clay on their hands. "That's how easily an STD can be transmitted," I told them.

"I made some bad choices in my life," I told that room full of five hundred students. "God forgave me for those choices. There are no literal 'do overs' for virginity, but you can have a new beginning from this moment in time forward. I had a new beginning once. Seven years later, I consecrated my relationship with my wife after we were married."

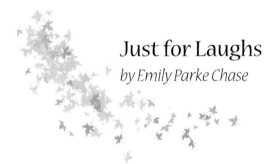

Just for Laughs

by Emily Parke Chase

A girl rushes into a room of students, waving a piece of bright pink paper, a love note from her boyfriend. Eagerly, she shares it with her two best friends:

> *Last night was amazing! Lying beside you, touching your soft skin . . . No one else can ever be all that you are to me, not today, not tomorrow, not ever. You rock my world!*
>
> *Love, Jeff*

Her two friends pull out identical pink pieces of paper from their pockets and wave them in the air too—copies of the exact same note!

Laughter erupts from the crowd watching. This was a skit, a part of our "Waiting: The Smart Choice!" abstinence education program that is presented in local schools throughout the capital region of Pennsylvania. Ninety percent of our presentations are in public schools.

When I first began serving as a volunteer at our local pregnancy center, I saw many clients who walked into our center for pregnancy tests. They carried heavy loads of fear, embarrassment, or anger, results of their decisions to become sexually active. Though our medical staff and advocates worked hard to restore the clients' sense of worth and help them make better choices in the future, I yearned to reach these young people before they became sexually active, before they were emotionally wounded.

From the very start, I desired to take into the schools a positive message of sexual self-control. Using skits, role plays, and a healthy dose of humor, I developed the "Waiting: The Smart Choice!" program. I wanted young people to understand that sexual intimacy is something exciting and worth saving for marriage.

To keep the program lively and up-to-date, I recruited college students from local campuses to assist as peer presenters. The first year we only had five students helping, but the following year we had about eighteen, and doors began opening into more schools. We did sixty programs that year and were elated. Then the numbers began to jump. We had thirty-eight young people sign up to help the next fall; the next year it was ninety-five. Soon over one hundred college students were volunteering to help with over three hundred programs each year!

High school students love to laugh. When we ask them what they are looking for in a dating relationship, a ninth grader may tell us the first thing he notices about a girl is her looks. In response to the comment, one of my college peer presenters races up to a student in the class and says, "You have the most beautiful nose in the world! I've got to be with that nose for the rest of my life. Will you marry me?" The class laughs as we illustrate how that relationship might change when the nose is broken. If the class still doubts that looks can change, we suggest they glance at their parents' high school yearbooks!

Instead of lecturing on sexual self-control, we ask questions: "How can you keep things from getting out of hand when you are out on a date? Suppose you are at the local miniature golf course. Is it probable that the couple ahead of you on the putting green will give in to a sudden urge to have sex and do it right there on the green in front of a crowd?" The class laughs. They get the point: it's easier to stay in control when other people are around.

But sometimes the joke is on us. One college student went into the hallway to grab a prop for the climax of a scene, only to find our crutch had disappeared. A practical joker had walked off with our prop.

At a church youth group, Chad was doing a skit that involved a piece of gum and two girls from the audience. He offered his lucky piece of gum to the first young woman as an expression of his love and commitment to the relationship, but when she bit into the gum, she made a horrible face. I realized that by mistake I had bought Sour Patch flavored gum! Frothing at the mouth, the girl spit it into a nearby wastebasket. Chad didn't bat an eye. He merely continued with the skit, approaching the second girl and professing his love for her. Again, as a symbol of his affection, he wanted to offer the new girl his special piece of gum, but he realized he needed to retrieve his gum from the first girl. He bent over the wastebasket, searched for the chewed gum and fished it out. Folding the gum into its original foil wrapper, he offered it to his new girlfriend. The teen audience laughed as the second girl turned him down in no uncertain terms, but the class got the message: Some things are more special the first time they are offered.

Evaluations from the high school students who hear our message always offer a source of entertainment. One student appreciated the concept of "renewed virginity," except she spelled it "re-nude virginity"! A male student wrote with great seriousness, "Now I know I'll be sterile until marriage." We decided he should marry the girl who commented on her evaluation, "I'll never have sex until I'm pregnant!"

While our colleagues at the pregnancy center mop up the tears caused by their clients' broken relationships and unplanned pregnancies, we who carry a message of sexual self-control into the schools offer a message of hope and see lives changed as we serve up a mixture of truth and laughter.

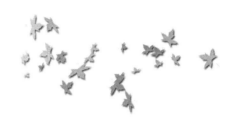

Resources

 Find helpful materials mentioned in the stories in chapter 9 here:
• Heartbeat International's "The Sexual Integrity Program" http://www.heartbeatservices.org/sexual-integrity/sexual-integrity-home
"Steps to Sexual Health" DVDs with Dr. Doug Weiss http://www.heartbeatservices.org/sexual-integrity/steps-to-sexual-health

 Find abstinence education materials here:
• International Life Services Abstinence Education Program:
http://www.internationallifeservices.org/abstinenceeducation.cfm or (800) 395-HELP
Abstinence Clearinghouse, http://www.abstinence.net/ or (605) 335-3643

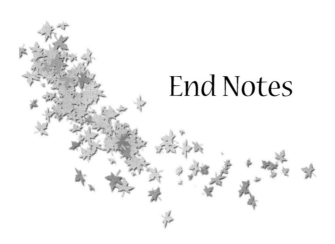

End Notes

Chapter 1: Who Faces Unplanned Pregnancy?

[1] "Facts on Induced Abortion in the United States," Guttmacher Institute* "In Brief," May 2010, 1. *The Guttmacher Institute was founded in 1968 as a semiautonomous division of The Planned Parenthood Federation of America. The organization was renamed in memory of Alan Guttmacher, a former president of Planned Parenthood and became an independent, not-for-profit corporation in 1977. ("Guttmacher Institute," Wikipedia, accessed 10/6/10, http://en.wikipedia.org/wiki/Guttmacher_Institute.)

[2] "Fertility, Family Planning, and Reproductive Health of U.S. Women: Data from the 2002 National Survey of Family Growth," U.S. Department of Health and Human Services, Centers for Disease Control and Prevention, National Center for Health Statistics, accessed 11/18/10, http://www.cdc.gov/nchs/data/series/sr_23/sr23_025.pdf, 13.

[3] "Fertility, Family Planning, and Reproductive Health," CDC, 13.

[4] "Facts on Induced Abortion," Guttmacher "In Brief," 1.

Chapter 2: What About Her Family?

[i] "Reported Legal Abortions by Age Group Within the State of Occurrence, 2006," Henry J. Kaiser Family Foundation, accessed 10/7/2010, http://www.statehealthfacts.org/faq.jsp. The Kaiser Family Foundation is a nonprofit, private operating foundation and is not associated with Kaiser Permanente or Kaiser Industries.

[2] "Abortion Facts," The Center for Bio-Ethical Reform, accessed 10/6/10, http://www.abortionno.org/Resources/fastfacts.html.

[3] "Get "In the Know:" 20 Questions About Pregnancy, Contraception and Abortion," Guttmacher Institute, accessed 7/11/07, http://www.guttmacher.org/in-the-know/index.html.

[4] "Recent Trends in Teenage Pregnancy in the United States, 1990–2002," U.S. Department of Health and Human Services, Centers for Disease Control and Prevention, National Center for Health Statistics, page last updated 4/6/10, http://www.cdc.gov/nchs/products/pubs/pubd/series/sr23/pre-1/sr23_25.htm.

[5] "Abortion Facts," Bio-Ethical Reform, 10/6/10.

[6] "Teen Birth Rates Rose Again in 2007, Declined in 2008," Centers for Disease Control and Prevention, page last reviewed 5/5/10, http://www.cdc.gov/features/dsteenpregnancy/.

Chapter 3: When a Woman Considers Abortion

[1] "Abortion Facts," The Center for Bio-Ethical Reform, accessed 10/6/10, http://www.abortionno.org/Resources/fastfacts.html.

[2] "Abortion Facts," Bio-Ethical Reform, 10/6/10.

Chapter 4: Learning from Those Who Have Experienced Abortion

[1] "Facts on Induced Abortion In the United States," Guttmacher Institute "In Brief," May 2010, 1.

[2] "Abortion's Psycho-Social Consequences," National Right to Life Educational Trust Fund, Washington, CD, accessed 11/18/10, http://www.nrlc.org/Factsheets/FS18_AbtnPsychoSocial.pdf.

[3] "Abortion Facts," The Center for Bio-Ethical Reform, accessed 10/6/10, http://www.abortionno.org/Resources/fastfacts.html.

[4] "Abortion Facts," Bio-Ethical Reform, 10/6/10.

[5] "Abortion: Some Medical Facts," National Right to Life Committee, accessed 10/6/10, http://www.nrlc.org/abortion/ASMF/asmf13.html.

[6] "Former Abortion Clinic Owner Carol Everett," Prolife Action League, accessed 10/6/10, http://www.prolifeaction.org/providers/everett.php.

[7] Lanfranchi, M.D., F.A.C.S., Angela, and Joel Brind, Ph.D. *Breast Cancer Risks and Prevention* Fourth Edition, (New York: Breast Cancer Prevention Institute, 2005, 2007), 8.

[8] "Abortion – Before, During, and After an Abortion: When to Call a Doctor," WebMD.com, accessed 7/19/07, http://women.webmd.com/tc/Abortion-Before-During-and-After-an-Abortion-When-to-Call-a-Doctor.

[9] "Placenta previa," WebMd.com, accessed 10/6/10, http://www.webmd.com/hw-popup/placenta-previa.

[10] "Abortion Facts," Bio-Ethical Reform, 10/6/10.

[11] "Facts on Induced Abortion," Guttmacher "In Brief," 1.

[12] "Abortion Facts," Bio-Ethical Reform, 10/6/10.

[13] "Get 'In the Know': Questions About Pregnancy, Contraception and Abortion," Guttmacher Institute, accessed 7/11/2007, www.guttmacher.org/in-the-know/characteristics.html.

[14] "Is Abortion Safe?: Psychological Consequences," National Right to Life Committee, accessed 10/6/10, http://www.nrlc.org/abortion/ASMF/asmf14.html.

[15] "Abortion Facts," Bio-Ethical Reform, 10/6/10.

[16] "Fertility, Family Planning, and Reproductive Health of U.S. Women: Data from the 2002 National Survey of Family Growth," U.S. Department of Health and Human Services, Centers for Disease Control and Prevention, National Center for Health Statistics, accessed 11/18/10, http://www.cdc.gov/nchs/data/series/sr_23/sr23_025.pdf, p. 13.

[17] "Facts on Induced Abortion," Guttmacher "In Brief," 1.

Chapter 5: For, By, and About Men

[1] "Abortion Facts," The Center for Bio-Ethical Reform, accessed 10/6/10, http://www.abortionno.org/Resources/fastfacts.html.

[2] "Post-Abortive Men," Ramah International, accessed 10/11/10, http://www.ramahinternational.org/for-post-abortive-men.html.

[3] "Facts on Induced Abortion In the United States," Guttmacher Institute "In Brief," May 2010, 1.

[4] "Abortion in the United States: Statistics and Trends," National Right to Life, accessed 10/7/10, http://www.nrlc.org/abortion/facts/abortionstats.html. Using estimates from both the Alan Guttmacher Institute and the Center for Disease Control, this site estimated the total number of abortions in the United States since *Roe v. Wade* in 1973 through 2007 at 49,551,703.

Chapter 6: Helping Her Keep Her Child

[1] "Abortion Facts," The Center for Bio-Ethical Reform, accessed 10/6/10, http://www.abortionno.org/Resources/fastfacts.html.

[2] "Fertility, Family Planning, and Reproductive Health of U.S. Women: Data from the 2002 National Survey of Family Growth," U.S. Department of Health and Human Services, Centers for Disease Control and Prevention, National Center for Health Statistics, accessed 11/18/10, http://www.cdc.gov/nchs/data/series/sr_23/sr23_025.pdf, p. 13.

[3] "Fertility, Family Planning, and Reproductive Health," CDC, 13.

Chapter 7: When a Woman Gives Her Child for Adoption

[1] Jones, Ph.D., Jo, "Who Adopts? Characteristics of Women and Men Who Have Adopted Children," NCHS Data Brief, no. 12, National Center for Health Statistics, 2009, 1.

[2] Jones, "Who Adopts?," 5.

[3] "Abortion Facts," The Center for Bio-Ethical Reform, accessed 10/6/10, http://www.abortionno.org/Resources/fastfacts.html.

[4] Jones, "Who Adopts?," 2.

[5] Jones, "Who Adopts?," 1, 5.

Chapter 8: Who Are These People Who Help Women Find Options?

[1] "Iowa PRC Receives First Ultrasound," Heartlink, accessed 4/27/04, http://www.family.org/pregnancy/ultrasound/a0031676.cfm.

[2] "About Care Net," Care Net, accessed 10/6/10, https://www.care-net.org/aboutus/.

[3] "The Basics," National Right to Life Committee, Factsheets (http://www.nrlc.org/Factsheets/index.html), accessed 10/710, http://www.nrlc.org/Factsheets/FS09_TheBasics.pdf.

[4] "Pain of the Unborn," National Right to Life Committee, Factsheets (http://www.nrlc.org/Factsheets/index.html), accessed 10/710, http://www.nrlc.org/abortion/Fetal_Pain/Fetal-Pain091604.pdf.

[5] "Our Leadership," Heartbeat International, accessed 10/6/10, http://www.heartbeatinternational.org/heartbeatint-about-us/our-leadership.

Chapter 9: Reaching Out, Helping People, and Preventing Unplanned Pregnancy

[1] "Steps to Sexual Health," Heartbeat International, accessed 8/3/10, http://www.heartbeatservices.org/sexual-integrity/steps-to-sexual-health.

Contributors

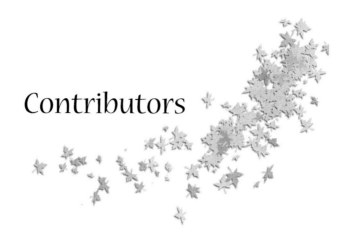

Lucy Neeley Adams is a speaker, singer, and storyteller. Her work at the crisis pregnancy center in Murfreesboro, Tennessee, was an extra blessing. Visit www.52hymns.com to read about her music ministry or purchase her book, *52 Hymn Story Devotions*, or purchases at any online bookstore.

Phyllis Allen resides in Colorado with her four children. She served as Executive Director of the Pregnancy Assistance League prior to its closing in 1998. A member of the American Association of Christian Counselors, Phyllis reaches out to hurting women and youth through her writing and her internet-based ministry.

Connie Ambrecht, with her husband, Dan, founded Sonography Now, an on-site ultrasound training company, in 2002. Additionally, together they founded Hope Imaging (www.hopeimaging.org), an organization that partners with medical missions for domestic and overseas ultrasound machine acquisition and training. Either together, or on solo trips, since 2005 Connie and Dan have taken their training to Armenia, Romania, Ukraine, Ecuador, Haiti, and the Philippines. Connie enjoys speaking with Dan at pregnancy center banquets whenever possible. www.truthlinknow.com

Dan Ambrecht, along with his wife, Connie, co-owns Sonography Now, a company that trains medical personnel to use ultrasound. The parent company, Truth Link Now, offers several other nonmedical training programs. Their organization, Hope Imaging, helps with ultrasound machine acquisition and training for both domestic and overseas medical missions. He and Connie enjoy speaking at pregnancy center banquets whenever possible. In his spare time, Dan is a test rider for Harley-Davidson at the Arizona Proving Ground. www.truthlinknow.com, www.hopeimaging.org

Sonja Bates teaches *SaveOne*, a post-abortion Bible study, through the church she attends, Judson Baptist Church in San Bernardino, California, and through the San Bernardino Pregnancy Resource Center. http://www.sbpcc.net/post-abortion_help.htm

Tina Brock has since married Darrell. They have two children. Since the healing from her abortion experience, she has shared her testimony many times and has been a guest on *The Faces of Abortion* television program. Tina recently completed a small book of poems from babies in the womb speaking to different people, titled *Whispers From The Womb*. www.whispersfromthewomb.com

Jade Chartier lives in Brighton, Colorado, with her husband, Bill, who is currently the Colorado State Coordinator for the Christian Motorcyclists Association (www.cmausa.org), and two dogs. Jade has three sons and eight grandchildren. Some of her favorite interests are motorcycling and reading and studying her Bible. She loves to spend time with her grandchildren and cuddling her dogs. She currently works for the district attorney of Adams County, Colorado.

Emily Parke Chase helped found the Capital Area Pregnancy Centers, Camp Hill, Pennsylvania. She has served there as a volunteer for over twenty years and developed their abstinence curriculum, *Waiting, The Smart Choice!* She is the author of *Why Say No When My Hormones Say Go?* Visit her at www.emilychase.com.

Janne Strobel Collins has worked for Sussex Pregnancy Care Center as Coordinator of Volunteers for the past ten years. She is coauthor of the *Good Health Cook Book: A Nutritional Approach to Wellness.* She and her husband Eric live in Delaware.

Erin Kiker Di Paolo is a freelance writer and employee of Frontier Airlines who currently lives in Denver, Colorado. She is a single mom of three children: Joseph, 18, James 16, and Alessandra 13 and the beloved girlfriend of Richard Dittman. She graduated with a degree in Journalism from Colorado State University in Fort Collins, Colorado, in 1985 and is passionate about writing, travel, sports, warm weather, and the beach.

Patrice Egging is a former member of the founding board of ABC Pregnancy Help Center in Pratt, Kansas, and former Director of ABC. She lives in Pratt, Kansas, with her husband Mike. They have six grown children and nine grandchildren. Using gifts of music she encourages those who need hope and healing. To contact Patrice about coming to your area, visit: Patrice Egging: Music and Ministry at http://patriceegging.com. E-mail her at mpegging@havilandtelco.com.

Ann Eppard lives with her family in Lakewood, Colorado.

Anita Estes is an art teacher and freelance writer. Her work appears in several publications including *God Allows U-Turns for Women* and *A Cup of Comfort Book of Prayer.* She has authored the book, *When God Speaks,* and compiled another about men freed from addictions, *Transformed: Inspiring Stories of Freedom.* Visit her website www.AnitaEstes.com.

Anne S. Grace, through Gift of Grace Ministries, writes inspirational articles and books. *Grace Upon Grace*, her journey of faith, is available from www.AuthorHouse.com. Anne is active at church, Aglow International, Women in Christian Media, and two writer's networks. She and her husband live near Hilton Head Island, South Carolina. They have four children and eight grandchildren. www.giftofgrace.injesus.com

Besides writing, **Helen Hoover** enjoys sewing, knitting, traveling, and walking in the mountains. Serving God as part of the Sower Ministry for retired Christian RVers is a fulfilling venture in her and her husband's lives. Word Aflame Publications, *The Secret Place*, Word Action publishing, *The Quiet Hour, The Lutheran Digest*, Light and Life Communications, and *Victory in Grace* have published her devotionals and personal articles.

Karie Hughes is an author, speaker, wife, mom, birthmom, and a "gigi" of two grandbabies. An enthusiastic and informed advocate, she is devoted to thinking about what the next generation needs and proactively moves on those needs every day with relevance and objectivity. Karie currently trains parents in homes, conferences, crisis pregnancy centers, etc., to be intentional in speaking about purity and teen sex. Contact her to schedule a presentation and training at your pregnancy center or church: 480.326.8990 karie@kariehughes.com www.passionandprinciples.blogspot.com

Chris Jackman is currently pursuing her love of Biblical Hebrew, writing songs from Scripture and singing them in Hebrew. www.ChrisJackman.com. Her CD, *The Choice,* is available through www.AbortionRecovery.org.

Karen Reno Knapp loves living in the Endless Mountains of Pennsylvania with her husband, John. She also enjoys writing, swimming, traveling, and playing her NBA fantasy team. She blogs about writing at www.KarenRenoKnapp.blogspot.com. Learn about her husband's writing at www.EarthIsNotAlone.com.

Rita Leone-Reyes began her journey in pro-life work as a pregnancy center volunteer in Audubon, New Jersey, in 1989 after experiencing her own unplanned pregnancy as a college student. In 1996 she cofounded and is presently the Executive Director of Choices of the Heart, serving two locations in South Jersey. Rita has spoken to hundreds at churches, banquets, retreats, and national seminars on women's issues, upholding the sanctity of life and sharing the gospel of Jesus Christ. She is married and the mother of three. www.ChoicesoftheHeart.com

Carol McGalliard is a freelance writer in Greensboro, NC. She is a member of Westover Church where she is team leader for Journey, a ministry to survivors of abuse. Carol is married to Ray, has two stepchildren and two grandchildren. In her spare time, Carol enjoys SCUBA, traveling, and art.

John T. McNeal has had over seventeen articles published at *TheChristianPulse.com* and has spent over ten years working with the Children's Ministry at Chestnut Mountain Church in Flowery Branch, Georgia. He is currently working on entering the ministry full-time and his first novel. Married with one son, he is happiest when he is serving the Lord. You can get in touch with John at: www.PrayerRock.org/ PrayerRock@hotmail.com

Barb Musso has served as Executive Director of A Caring Pregnancy Center in Pueblo, Colorado, for seven years and Client Services Director the seven years prior. After college she worked with unwed teen mothers and adoption services through Catholic Charities in Pueblo, and later worked with teens in a Christian school. She raised two daughters with her husband Don. Barb says, "Leading others to Christ through the truth of God's Word can help people far more than any program available."

Shirley A. Reynolds is a freelance writer living in the mountains of Idaho. Not only is writing her passion, but hiking the back trails, riding her ATV, taking pictures of the beautiful mountain scenery, and learning to live a country life, as compared with being raised in a big city atmosphere. She can be reached by e-mail at <u>heartprints@netzero.com</u>.

Marcia Samuels* is now retired. She received her pregnancy center training from the Christian Action Council. Her experience includes working for the Kansas City Youth for Christ at the Lighthouse (a ministry for abortion-risk girls). She has also served as a Director of a crisis pregnancy center she helped to open.

Marilyn M. Scott has been the executive director of the Pregnancy Crisis Center in Twin Falls, Idaho, for the past twenty-two years. She has been married thirty years to her wonderful and supportive husband Kelly. She has three children: Hailey is twenty-two and sons Jordan and Jameson are nineteen. She sees each new client as a new opportunity to serve Christ and believes each day is a gift God gives us—what we do with it is our gift to Him.

Jami Sims is a wife to her husband Brad, mother to their eight blessings: Madelyn, James, Sydney, Riley, Sara Joy, Bo, Carrie, and little numero ocho, Joel, came in June 2010. If you are looking for a speaker for a ladies' event, Pregnancy Resource Center fund-raising banquet, Sanctity of Human Life service, or anything in between, book Jami today: <u>jamisims@gmail.com</u> or 334.319.2561.

George Sluppick still rides his Harley, fishes, writes music, and plays bass in the church band besides all the necessary work of maintaining his and his wife, Judy's, home. He says, "Even though I'm retired, I rarely find myself with a lot of free time!"

 224

Judy Sluppick was born and raised in Natchitoches, Louisiana. After teaching for 27 years, she retired to help husband, George, with their Christian bookstore. She volunteered at the local crisis pregnancy center and later became the Executive Director of the Women's Resource Center for 13 years before retiring. She recently said, "I started a dance ministry at our church that I enjoy so much."

Kyleen Stevenson-Braxton is a published writer and speaker. She is part owner of Fashion Crossroads, Inc., in Casper, Wyoming, and is married with two adopted children. Kyleen served as the post-abortion healing coordinator for Care Net Pregnancy and Resource Clinic of Casper for five years and helped many others receive the same healing she found through a post-abortion recovery class. She shares her story publically and is currently working on a book titled *Barren* which recounts her journey through abortion, infertility, and adoption. Learn more at http://singobarrenwoman.wordpress.com. Contact her at braxtonk@bresnan.net.

Kelly Stigliano lives in Orange Park, Florida, with her husband Jerry. Kelly is a freelance writer, reporter, and speaker, touching hearts everywhere with her testimony. She and Jerry volunteer weekly at First Coast Women's Services in Clay County, Florida. To learn more check out www.kellystigliano.com.

Connie Suarez has found in pregnancy center ministry the perfect venue to be an advocate for the unborn and those still needing to find a Savior. The Arkansas Valley Pregnancy Center in La Junta, Colorado, has been her passion for over fifteen years. In her spare time, Connie loves to read and write. Learn more at www.conniesuarez.com.

Joyce Sykes lives in North Carolina with David, her husband. She is blessed with three children and four beautiful granddaughters. Her heart's desire is to continue to touch the hearts of the women who the Lord places in her path.

225

Pamela S. Thibodeaux, an award-winning author, is the cofounder and a lifetime member of Bayou Writers Group in Lake Charles, Louisiana, and a member of White Roses in Bloom Authors. Multipublished in romantic fiction as well as creative nonfiction, her writing has been tagged as, "Inspirational with an edge!" and reviewed as "steamier and grittier than the typical Christian novel *without* decreasing the message." http://www.pamelathibodeaux.com http://pamswildroseblog.blogspot.com http://whiterosesinbloom.blogspot.com

Sue Tornai, the author of more than sixty articles and stories, lives with her husband, John, and dog, Maggie, in Carmichael, California. Sue has invested twenty years of her life in the next generation by teaching elementary Sunday school. She writes stories for children, devotions, and magazine articles. Sue blogs at: www.missue.blogspot.com, www.suetornai.wordpress.com, and http://pathwaysonline.net. Her website is www.suetornai.com.

JoAnn Valdez has been the director of Hope Pregnancy Center in Trinidad, Colorado, for eighteen years. She lives with her husband in Trinidad.

Brittany Valentine considers her most precious identity in life to be that of a child of God (John 1:12). She is passionate about the call of God on her life to encourage Bible literacy and application within the body of believers. She is available to speak to ladies groups on a variety of topics. Please visit her blog at www.purposedperspective.wordpress.com to study the Word along with her.

Scotty Vaughn is the "crazy" one of the critically acclaimed "Colorado Cowboys for Jesus," one of the premier cowboy gospel groups in the country. After twenty-nine years as the resident emcee and storyteller at the world famous "Flying W

Ranch" in Colorado Springs, Colorado, he answered God's call to ministry and became senior pastor at the Church on the Ranch at the Flying W Ranch. He is the founder of "Cowboy Up," a men's outreach of Life Network. www.churchontheranch.org

Bonnie Watkins has taught ages 2 to 92 in high school, community college, GED prep, SAT prep, English as a Second Language (ESL), writing workshops, Bible studies, and Sunday school. She and husband Dan live in Austin, Texas. She has two married sons and now, two daughters (their wives). Stay tuned for grandchildren.

Joyce Zounis moved from being a client to a volunteer and then onto a pregnancy resource center director in Colorado. She has hosted and produced Operation Outcry's radio show, *Voices of Abortion*, and TV show, *Faces of Abortion*. She is featured in the 2007 documentary *I Was Wrong* with Norma McCorvey, "Jane Roe" in the landmark Supreme Court case *Roe v. Wade*. Joyce produces and hosts *Beyond the Bandaide™ Radio* which can be heard daily on National ProLife Radio. Her story is also featured in the 2010 released DVD, *Life After Abortion*. http://www.voicesoftruth.net/ http://www.lifeafterabortion.info/

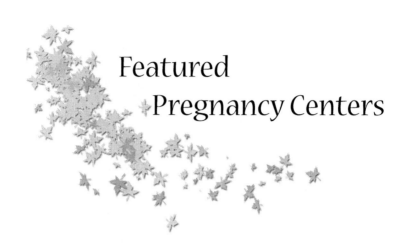

Featured Pregnancy Centers

ABC Pregnancy Help Center in Pratt, Kansas, featured in Patrice Egging's story, is now the **Pratt Family Life Center.**

A Caring Pregnancy Center was incorporated as Pueblo Crisis Pregnancy Center in 1984 and changed to A Caring Pregnancy Center in 1992. Services offered included free pregnancy tests with peer counseling, maternity and baby supplies, and parenting classes. In 2006 ACPC expanded to include ACPC Women's Clinic directly across the street, which offers pregnancy testing, ultrasound, and limited STI (sexually transmitted infections) testing and treatment. ACPC is currently working to reach Pueblo's college community. Pueblo has one of the highest teen pregnancy rates in Colorado. http://www.acpcpueblo.org/home.html

Arkansas Valley Pregnancy Center in La Junta, Colorado, opened to clients in 1995 and waited a month and a half for the first client. Today they average sixty clients per month. Each client has her own set of challenges and the staff and volunteers understand that they cannot meet her needs, but they know who can, so they patiently wait for an opportunity to introduce clients to Him, the Lord Jesus Christ. http://www.avpclj.org/

Birthright, where Anne S. Grace once worked, has moved but is located in Woodbridge, Virginia.

First Care Boca Raton, formerly Tender Loving Care (TLC) Pregnancy Center of Boca Raton featured in Joyce Zounis's story, is now one of a network of First Care Family Resources in Florida. First Care celebrated its 25-year anniversary in 2010. http://www.first-care.org/

Bridgeway is a loving home in Lakewood, Colorado, for pregnant teenagers, ages 16 to 21, providing support and education for the young women who come to live here. We offer an opportunity for these women to begin a new life of self-sufficiency, success, and happiness for themselves and their babies. We support our residents whether they choose parenting or an adoption plan. www.bridgewayhomes.org

The **Capital Area Pregnancy Centers** of Camp Hill, Pennsylvania, were founded in 1986 and offer a full range of confidential client services, including pregnancy testing, sonograms, limited STD testing, post-abortion support, and abstinence education programs. Visit them at www.lifechoicesclinic.org.

Care Net Pregnancy and Resource Clinic of Casper, Wyoming, is a Christian, life-affirming service organization providing emotional, spiritual, and material support to women and families dealing with an unplanned pregnancy. We educate about abortion procedures as well as the emotional, physical, and spiritual effects of abortion. It is our goal to see women healed from the sorrow and guilt that often follows abortion. We also offer confirmation of pregnancy using ultrasound and limited STD testing and treatment. All of our services are free of charge. www.carenetcasper.com www.carenetpartner.com

CareNet Pregnancy Center of NEPA has been operating in Susquehanna County, Pennsylvania, for ten years, after starting in Wyoming County twenty-five years ago. The Care Net Center of Hallstead, Pennsylvania, is now located in Montrose, the county seat, due to a flood in 2006.

Choices of the Heart, a woman's resource center, is one of the largest pregnancy centers in New Jersey serving two locations in South Jersey. In 2008, Choices became the nation's first pregnancy center offering ultrasound services in a shopping mall. Director Rita Leone-Reyes developed C.O.P.E.S. (Coalition of Pregnancy Emergency Services), an association developed to link pregnancy resource centers in New Jersey. www.ChoicesoftheHeart.com

First Care Boca Raton, formerly Boca Raton Tender Loving Care (TLC) Pregnancy Center featured in Joyce Zounis's story, is now one of a network of First Care centers in Florida. First Care celebrated its 25-year anniversary in 2010. http://www.first-care.org/

First Coast Women's Services (www.fcws.org) serves women and men in northeast Florida at four locations. FCWS offers truthful information, emotional support, and practical assistance to those facing unplanned pregnancies. They also provide opportunity for healing and restoration to those hurt by abortion. All services are free and confidential. Se habla español.

Franklin Life Crisis Pregnancy Center was opened in 2002 as a branch office of Toccoa Life, Inc. It was a dream-come-true for **Tina Brock**. She wanted to be there for women who may find themselves in an unexpected pregnancy just as she did after high school. Today, Tina is the Executive Director of Franklin Life Pregnancy Resource Center, Inc., in Carnesville, Georgia. www.franklinlifeprc.webs.com

Gainesville Care Center, featured in John McNeal's story, offers confidential and complimentary one-on-one support services to those facing a crisis pregnancy, STD health issues, and post-abortion trauma in a compassionate, Christian atmosphere. We proactively educate middle though college age students with the purity until marriage message. GCC partners with churches, agencies and other institutions, and all of our services are complimentary. Gainesville Care Center educates people to make godly sexual decisions and ministers the hope and love of Christ by saving lives and changing lives. www.GainesvilleCare.org

Hope Pregnancy Center in Trinidad, Colorado, offers an eight-week infant care program for new moms, a post-abortion support group to men and women, and W.A.I.T. (Why Am I Tempted!), a two-day abstinence program for 7th, 8th, and 9th grade students. They provide donated clothing, furniture, and baby items free to their clients. This center's mission is "to help new mothers successfully care for and raise their babies."

The Austin Crisis Pregnancy Center, featured in Bonnie Watkins's story, began in the 1980s and later changed its name to **LifeCare**. It continues to minister to women's spiritual and physical needs with free pregnancy tests, sonograms, counseling, maternity and children's clothes, birth and parenting classes, PALS programs, abstinence education in schools, and unconditional love.

Life Line Crisis Pregnancy Center, featured in Joyce Sykes's story "Life Line," has been a blessing and lifesaving instrument in God's master plan. Countless lives have been touched by the staff and volunteers throughout the years.

Lighthouse Ministries, Inc., 180 Lighthouse Lane, Reeves, Louisiana http://lighthouseministriesinc.org Visitors welcome. You may send donations to P.O. Box 130, Reeves, LA 70658. Patsy Cavenah 337-666-2678 patlite@centurytel.net

Living Well was founded in 1985. Living Well Medical Clinic in Orange, California, is a nonprofit, nonpolitical organization that is committed to serving women, men, teens, parents, and all those involved in a circumstance where a pregnancy is unplanned or unwanted. Their goal is to meet the physical, emotional, and spiritual needs of those seeking help. http://www.living-well.org/

New Hope Adoptions Services featured in Shirley A. Reynolds's story, "The LifeSavers®," helped young women facing unscheduled pregnancies by offering counseling, financial help, family support, and home visits. New Hope Family Services is no longer in operation; it combined with Bethany Adoption Services in Seattle, Washington.

New Paltz Pregnancy Support Center featured in Anita Estes's story, "The Right Choice," changed its name to **The Pregnancy Support Center of Ulster County**, which upholds the value of human life by befriending, comforting, and supporting those with pregnancy-related needs. They offer God's love by proclaiming the Gospel of Christ and His plan for sexuality, marriage, and the family to their community.

Pregnancy Crisis Center in Twin Falls, Idaho, opened in 1979. It has grown from a one-room office in the Salvation Army basement to a beautiful full-service pregnancy help center with plans to become medical soon. Annually, the center serves nearly 600 crisis clients, 1500 through the pregnancy and parenting classes, and another 1500 through abstinence classes.

San Bernardino Pregnancy Resource Center offers many free services, including the *SaveOne* class Sonja Bates taught. http://www.sbpcc.net/

Sussex Pregnancy Care Center, represented in Janne Strobel Collins's story, is currently celebrating its twenty-fifth year of life-saving services in Sussex County, Delaware.

Tender Loving Care (TLC) Pregnancy Center of Boca Raton featured in Joyce Zounis's story is now First Care Boca Raton, one of a network of First Care Family Resources in Florida. First Care celebrated its 25-year anniversary in 2010. http://www.first-care.org/

Turning Point Women's Resource Center became a reality in Bergenfield, New Jersey, in October 2002 and has touched the lives of over 400 women. For eight years we operated on gifts of churches and individuals with no paid staff. In 2010 Turning Point begins a new chapter as we are absorbed by Lighthouse, a larger center, will move to a nearby city, and add ultrasound to our services. Our new location will afford us greater opportunities to serve women in unplanned pregnancies. http://www.lighthouseprc.org/

Women's Resource Center in Natchitoches, Louisiana, featured in Judy and George Sluppick's stories, opened in 1989 to give women hope by sharing the love of Christ, reach abortion-minded and vulnerable clients, and give alternatives to abortion to help women choose life for their babies. In 2006, WRC became a medical clinic adding two nurses, an ultrasound, and STD testing. Since 2008, they are a Life Choice Project enabling them to see clients longer and build closer relationships with them.

Dianne E. Butts served on the board of directors for a pregnancy center and in that time witnessed many courageous, life-changing stories. It has become her passion to help people share their stories of unplanned pregnancy so others can avoid regrets, find healing for past regrets, and locate practical resources.

A writer for twenty years, Dianne is the author of *Dear America: A Letter of Comfort and Hope to a Grieving Nation*. She has contributed to 17 books, has over 250 articles and short stories published in print magazines, and is an aspiring screenwriter. Her short film screenplay, *A Cowboy's Faith*, inspired by Scotty Vaughn's story in this book, was a finalist in the 168 Film Project's 2010 "Write of Passage" contest and will be produced as a short film soon.

Dianne lives with her husband in Colorado.
Visit her web sites and blog at:
www.DeliverMeBook.com,
www.DeliverMeBook.blogspot.com,
www.DianneEButts.com.

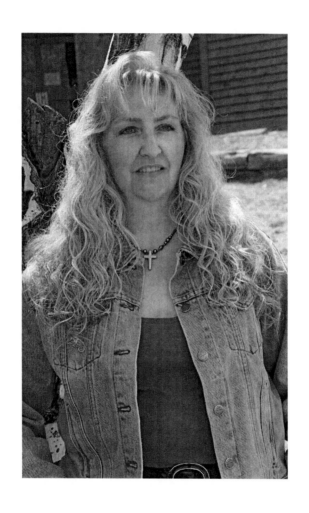

9 780983 164906